IN OUR
SUFFERING,
LORD
BE NEAR

PRAYERS OF
HOPE FOR THE
HURTING

BEN LOCKE

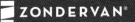

ZONDERVAN®

ZONDERVAN

In Our Suffering, Lord Be Near

© 2024 by Ben Locke

Published in Grand Rapids, Michigan, by Zondervan. Zondervan is a registered trademark of The Zondervan Corporation, L.L.C., a wholly owned subsidiary of HarperCollins Christian Publishing, Inc.

Requests for information should be addressed to customercare@harpercollins.com.

ISBN 978-0-310-46523-2 (audiobook)
ISBN 978-0-310-46516-4 (eBook)
ISBN 978-0-310-46511-9 (HC)

Cover design: Tiffany Forrester

Interior design: Emily Ghattas

Printed in Malaysia

24 25 26 27 28 COS 10 9 8 7 6 5 4 3 2 1

Contents

A Note to the Reader   v

Preface   viii

PART 1. FROM CRISIS TO SAFETY   1
Our prayers in crisis as God offers us safety

PART 2. FROM DESPAIR TO LAMENT   27
Our prayers of despair as God invites us to honest, raw lament

PART 3. FROM DEFIANCE TO SUBMISSION   47
Our prayers of defiance as God invites us to submit to Him

PART 4. FROM GRIEF TO RESCUE   63
Our prayers of grief as God offers to be our rescue

PART 5. FROM WANDERING TO OBEDIENCE   87
Our prayers in wandering as God invites us to be obedient to Him

PART 6. FROM CROSSROADS TO JUSTICE   107
Our prayers at a crossroads as God reveals His justice and truth

PART 7. FROM RESILIENCE TO STRENGTH 121
Our prayers of resilience and movement as God gives us strength

PART 8. FROM REDEMPTION TO DELIVERANCE 143
Our prayers of redemption as God delivers us into His forgiveness

PART 9. FROM PRAISE TO ADOPTION 167
Our prayers of praise as God adopts us as His beloved children

In Closing   186
A Final Charge   188
Acknowledgments   190
About the Author   192

A Note to the Reader

Sister, Brother, Mother, Father, Husband, Wife, Child, Friend, Warrior, My Fellow Sufferer—

You are not alone. You are not forgotten, nor are you overlooked. You are not too broken, nor are you too far gone. You are not crazy, nor are you defeated. There is breath still in your lungs; therefore there is absolute purpose for your life.

Thank the Lord, it is undoubtedly true.

My invitation as you read this book is simple: come as you are. Don't fake a single thing. Approach every word with absolute vulnerability and honesty, and don't withhold even an ounce of your emotion. If you are bitter, bring your bitterness. If you are angry, bring your anger. If you are sad, bring your sadness. If you are empty, bring your emptiness. Bring your tears, groans, cries for help—bring it all. Come as you are with the fullness of what you are carrying.

All I ask is that you come with the right expectation. But do not come with the expectation that this book is going to solve your problems, or that reciting a prayer will give you the miracle you've been waiting for. Come with the expectation that the God of the universe cares infinitely for you and is unequivocally listening to your every word and your every emotion. His presence is the reward we are after. That's it. With this posture, the gift we receive is not an outcome, a change of circumstance, or an answer to prayer we can touch or see. The gift is *Him*—*His* promises, *His* grace, *His* plans, *His* will.

Come as you are, as you *really* are—every wound, every sin, every emotion, every piece of your humanity. But come earnestly with the expectation that God alone will give you everything you need. Seek Him with the understanding that He is seeking you. Pray to Him knowing He is listening and acting, regardless of what you may see or not see, feel or not feel.

My promise to you is that your pursuit will not be in vain. If you give Him everything you have—good and bad, earnestly and with expectation—He will redeem you in your suffering. He will restore you in your sorrows. He will give you life.

So, I invite you to join me in praying each of these words honestly and boldly:

> Here I am, O Lord;
> all of me,
> before all of You,
> here I am.
>
> I have nothing to give You
> but everything that I am,
> all that I carry,
> and a desperate hope
> that You will save me.
>
> Because all else has failed me,
> here I am.
> Because suffering brought me to ruins,
> here I am.

I will seek You
when I can barely move;
I will call out to You
when I can hardly breathe.
For I know
You are my only hope.

O Lord,
You are certain to deliver me,
for I am Your beloved.

Expectantly,
earnestly,
and without ceasing,
I will remain at Your feet.

You are all that I need;
here I am,
here I always will be.

Amen.

Preface

Suffering is the most important experience we have in this life. It may not be the best thing we experience, and it certainly isn't the most enjoyable, but it is undoubtedly the most important. If you picked up this book, you might already know that.

I'm sorry for whatever brought you to choose a book on suffering. However, I am also glad that you are here, and I believe you're in the right place. I celebrate that you are still standing, fighting, surviving, and pressing on. My desire is to share in whatever you are facing, have faced, or will face soon through the words in this book.

This is not something I wrote from me to you, standing on the other side of suffering, saying, "Keep your head up!" It is a magnifying glass on a particularly excruciating chapter of my life, as well as a telescope that reflects who I am today, a truthful extension of my heart, mind, body, and soul right now, right alongside you. I am next to you, shoulder to shoulder, hand in hand, whether you are barely standing, crawling on your knees, or struggling to get out of bed.

In many ways, this is not really a book at all. It is an invitation to share life's most miserable, challenging, and difficult experiences together. It's an honest glimpse into my personal suffering, yes, but it's also a tool that I hope you can use as you navigate through your own life. I hope that if you share some of these same emotions, you'll know you aren't alone. I hope this book helps you put words to your own suffering. I hope it forces you to confront the deepest and most honest parts of yourself, challenging you to bring those things to the Lord. Most of all, I hope it brings you closer to your Creator.

———

For a long time I hated my story. The challenges of what I was facing seemed unfair, and I felt ready to give up. I was at my breaking point when the Lord found me, saved me, and I began to write. Here's a glimpse of how this book came to be.

In the fall of 2019, my senior year of college, I was playing in an NCAA Division I soccer playoff game. It was a cold and windy November night in New Jersey as our team took the field for a must-win game. I was hoping to pursue a professional soccer career after I graduated, but I didn't know if it was possible. We ended up losing the game with ten seconds left on the clock. It was a devastating loss, and it made my future seem even more uncertain.

Two weeks later, I suddenly found myself in the emergency room. On the day after Thanksgiving, I was out to dinner with my family—my favorite people in the world. We were sitting in the restaurant when my body started to, for lack of a better term, "go weak." The floor began moving and the walls started spinning. I excused myself to the restroom and splashed cold water on my face, then returned to the table and acted as if nothing was wrong. But I couldn't hide my maladies for long; my body began shutting down, and I was quickly taken to the hospital.

I was placed in a bed in a crowded hallway, since there weren't any private rooms left. My condition became worse; my body felt like it was slipping in and out of consciousness, as if the lights were getting ready to turn off and never come back on again. In between tests and evaluations, I tried standing up from my hospital bed in hopes this might keep my systems alert. My head still felt like it was spinning, my body felt disconnected from my mind, and I thought I might die. After sitting in the hallway of the ER for what felt like an eternity, a doctor came to me with a message that is now the headline of my life: "We know something's wrong, but we have no idea what it is."

My life turned upside down after that trip to the ER. I spent the following months unable to get out of bed. Each day since, I have battled a slew of disorienting, life-draining, highly complex symptoms that stem from severe neurological damage caused by multiple severe brain traumas—concussions from playing sports and also an automobile accident—and a chronic autoimmune disease. Not a moment has gone by since without intense discomfort and pain. My dream of playing professional soccer was—is—over.

I was passed from doctor to doctor, diagnosis to diagnosis, each one different from the last. I had every scan, test, and lab the human body is capable of. I was drowning in depression, overwhelmed with emptiness, and paralyzed by anxiety. It felt like my life was ending.

I cursed God. I questioned how He could possibly be listening to me. I denounced His existence. I separated from the church because I felt too damaged, too broken to be part of that body. I saw myself as unqualified to worship God because I was too angry, bitter, and lonely. The church seemed too perfect, too put together to want a burdened person like me. Not only did it feel like my life was ending, but I was ready for it to end. I didn't recognize myself anymore, and I felt there was nothing left for me to give. I had no hope, no will, no desire to carry on.

Then, on the recommendation of my family, I decided to order a notebook. They had been telling me for months that I should write. "It might help," they'd say, and I would roll my eyes at how absurd that sounded. *They don't get it,* I thought. But eventually I caved and decided to do it. *The worst that could happen is that I might never use it,* I thought, *and I'd be out five dollars.* But shortly after the notebook showed up, it started gathering dust in my closet. I chose to ignore it.

Until one day, full of agony and anger, I picked it up and started to write.

From the moment I put pen to paper, I knew exactly who I wanted to write to: God. He was the target of all my bitterness, rage, disappointment, judgment, and condemnation. Of course, I was upset with other people and other things, but God had watched me get sick. He'd watched me as my life and my future slipped through my fingers. My soccer career was over. I'd lost friends. I struggled to get out of bed every morning and felt like I had no reason to live. He hadn't given me any relief, any answers, or any way out of my suffering. He didn't care, and I was going to make sure He knew what I had to say to Him.

Silly me.

What followed from that moment is what you'll see in the pages of this book. This is a snapshot of my interactions with God as I walked through the hardest moments of my life. Yes, they were and are formatted as prayers. But they are more than that:

They are tears.

They are words that I screamed alone in my room.

They are representations of and responses to intense moments of complete darkness.

These words capture moments when I wanted my life to end. Moments when I couldn't escape excruciating pain. Moments of loss. Moments of depression, anxiety, fear, shame, guilt, hopelessness, rage—the valleys of emotion.

These words are also joy.

They are moments of total and complete worship. Moments of clarity, redemption, and forgiveness. Experiences of God's providence, love, and perfect grace. Happiness, freedom, peace, contentment, fullness of understanding—the mountaintops of emotion.

These prayers are responses to God's Word. They are my own reflections of how, in my desperation, I experienced His Word come alive to me.

Prayer and Scripture help us experience the presence of God in many ways. There were some moments when I would pour out my heart in prayer, and I felt like I heard the promises I've read over and over in Scripture come back to me through gentle words; I imagined how God would whisper them over me if we ever had a traditional conversation between the two of us. These reminders of God's Word, steady and reassuring, are so meaningful to me; I felt like I had to share them with you. Throughout the book you'll see these moments when I imagined God speaking the promises of Scripture captured in italics.

As you read, I ask you to remember one important truth: at the end of the day, I am a sinner. I am not God; therefore my own feelings, perceptions, and thoughts do not trump His Word. They never should, and they never will. Without His Word and His instruction, prayer is meaningless and empty. I rejoice in the fact that we don't have to depend on ourselves for answers; the Lord has already given to us everything we need.

What you may not see, but I hope you'll understand, is how and why these words were written. Many of these prayers were written while on my knees, slumped over my bed because I wasn't able to sit upright in a chair. Many were written as tears were coming down my face or when my cheeks flushed red with anger. Each one came as a result of intense suffering. As God continued to humble me, I realized I shouldn't hold back from Him. *Why wouldn't I say what I'm really thinking if He knows exactly what's in my head and what's on my heart?*

So that's what I did.

Each excerpt embodies the fullness of a particular day, experience, emotion, affliction, or challenge. They are unfiltered, raw, and honest. And I think we owe that to God. He made us, He knows us, and He loves us, so why would we withhold from Him? Not only do we owe it to God, but this process is healing for us as His elected children. Our Father created us to feel, process, and be vulnerable, and there is something wonderfully intimate and healing that happens when we do those things in His presence. I'm not suggesting you curse God when something bad happens, but I am suggesting that you approach Him honestly, openly, and without reservation. Because I know He can handle it. He knows how to listen. He knows how to humble. He knows how to forgive. He knows how to respond.

Each prayer was written in a little graph-paper notebook. And after months of writing, I lost track of it; I forgot that I had given it to my sister. A few months later, she moved to a different state. Then I moved to a different house. Then I moved again. Then, almost a year later, as I was in bed and ready to fall asleep, I thought about the notebook. I reached out to her and asked if she knew where it was; I assumed it had been thrown out or left behind. But sure enough, that notebook had made it onto a shelf in her new apartment. Across state lines, through U-Haul trucks and moving boxes, somehow it had stuck around. She gave it back to me, and I kept on writing.

This notebook shouldn't exist.

And yet, it does. Now, my desire is to share it with you.

Experiencing the intensity of suffering, not running from it, revealed a lot about who I was. I learned that I didn't really know the Lord when I told myself I did. I was exposed for having a weak faith that disappeared when life got hard. I saw that God was an asset to me when life was good and a terror to me when life was bad. And when I finally realized these things about myself, my suffering started to become something I was grateful for. Sickness became a way to test my faith. Pain became a way to rely more and more on God's strength. Difficulty humbled me to the point where I finally began to understand just how broken I am and just how extreme my need is for a Redeemer.

To be clear, this process was—and still is—anything but smooth. I still yell and kick and throw tantrums at the Lord. I weep when the reality of my sickness and its effects on my body over-whelms me. I have anger in my heart that erupts in some moments, and I feel out of control in others. I am far from a finished product. Incredibly far. Impossibly far.

But now I know Jesus—like, *really* know Him—not just on Sundays. I know Him not because life is good or because it's convenient, but because life got impossibly hard—because I was confronted with my inability, brokenness, weakness, and insur-mountable pride. And that, dear friend, was a blessing.

I hope these prayers meet you in your own moments, whatever they may be and whatever you may be up against. Maybe you've lost a loved one, or you're battling an illness. Maybe you're overcome with depression, or you're fighting addiction. Maybe you're anxious, afraid, or wandering through life without direction. These words are not just prayers. They're cries for help, explosions of anger, mourning, weeping, grieving, celebrating, rejoicing, and praising. And I hope you use them that way. I hope you read these words and hear yourself speak. I hope they bring you to your knees, encouraging you to confess your insufficiency and beckoning you to express your most genuine emotions.

The Lord knows you. He sees your heart and He is ready to respond. Don't hide from Him, don't withhold from Him, and don't think the distance between your pain and His grace is too far. He can handle whatever you are fighting. So tell Him.

PART 1

FROM

CRISIS TO

SAFETY

We . . .
receive the news
get the call
are given the diagnosis
which leads to . . .
crisis.

The waves of death swirled about me; the
torrents of destruction overwhelmed me.
(2 Samuel 22:5)

He . . .
who knows all things
who is sovereign over all
who does all things for His perfect purposes
calls us into . . .
the safety of His presence.

Then You spoke.
My entire body trembled,
but my spirit rejoiced:

Sweet child,
My beloved creation,
you are mine.
Your spirit belongs to the army of angels,
the Heavenly host.
It cannot be overcome by pain and suffering;
it will never fade away,
nor will it rot into the ground.

I have drawn a line around you,
I have told the deceiver,
"This far you may go,
and no further."
For you belong to the assembly of the victorious,
to the side of Life,
which can never be taken from you.

Do you not see
that if it were your time to depart,
you would be no more?
Yet here you stand;
you have been sustained with the rising of the
  morning sun.

You have breath in your lungs,
truth has come to your rescue,
because it is truth in My name.

After you have suffered a little while,
I myself will restore, confirm, strengthen,
and establish you.
From that day forward,
you will never depart from Me.
You will be tested, shaken, beaten,
but you will not depart from your Almighty Father.

For you are My beloved,
My sweet, sweet child,
you whom I created,
who were dead to sin,
but are now alive in Christ.

In You, my soul finds rest, O Lord.
I see peace when I look upon Your face.
I know comfort because You know me.
Be gone, evil;
death, you are not welcome here.

Amen.

2

Shattered,
I bring myself to the foot of the throne.
Piece by piece,
I drag all that I have to the Father.
With my last ounce of energy,
I fall at the feet of my King.
I cannot lift my head;
I cannot raise a finger.
Wholly imperfect,
all that I have is a broken spirit.

This is me, Father.
All that I have,
I give to You.
All that I am is Yours.
In this world,
I have nothing.
In this body,
I have no hope.
But in you, O Lord,
I will carry on.

For I see now, so clearly,
that I am a foreigner,
a traveler in a place that is not my home.
If this were my home,
I would not wish to stay here.

But my home is in Your arms, O God,
my shelter is in Your presence.
My refuge is Your right hand,
my comfort is in Your light.

I am an infant,
a wanting child,
full of tears and need,
of which I cannot fulfill on my own.

So here I lie.
To be in Your presence is all that I want,
to be close,
to be near
to my Almighty Father.
Scoop me up in Your strong and mighty hands;
bring me close, so I can feel Your warmth.
Wrap me up in Your robes;
hold me tight.

Here is where I wish to be,
so here I will stay.
Silent, in solitude,
I will have all that I need if I am here with You.

Amen.

3

My life is a foreign concept to me.
My coming and going—
neither provides me with a clue.
Backward is forward,
left is right.
I am hopelessly directionless.

Each day is consumed by discomfort.
I spend my nights motionless,
yet rest evades me.
I cannot find any clarity for my mind,
my spirit longs for a path forward.
But days have turned to weeks,
weeks have become months,
and still I find no opportunity to walk through an open door.

I am torn between rest and stagnation,
faith and foolishness,
trust and pride.
My soul has ceased to envision a future;
my spirit has lost its ability to hope.
Everything I am longs to be made whole,
yet my moments are filled with brokenness.

I cannot escape this life of paralysis.

Amen.

4

Night and day,
I call on the Lord.
Morning, noon, and evening,
I lift my broken voice to God.
I bring my distress to the throne.
I lay my afflictions at the feet of the Almighty;
my voice grows hoarse with desperation.
Lowly, I bring my aching body into Your courts.

I am empty.
I have nothing left to give,
but that which You see—
a body covered with scars,
from my head to my toes,
a soul that has been overcome with suffering.
I cannot stand on my own.
Surely if I tried,
my legs could not sustain me,
my bones would cry out in despair.

Yet You raise my head in the morning.
The light of the sun fills my room;
Your mercy causes me to wake.
Pain engulfs me;
though I am trapped in the storm of its embrace,
You hold me still.
Your strength holds my head above the waters,
without You, the waves would take me under;
I would disappear from the earth.

But, my God,
You hold me still.

Therefore, I will press on.
I will continue to fight the good fight
for as long as You give me breath.
I will dwell with You in every moment;
I will seek Your face.
For I know nothing else will suffice;
I know every other option will fall short.

Sustain me, Father.
Keep my head above the water,
restore my body and my soul,
establish Your kingdom through my hands.
If not this,
take me away.
Remove me from this earth,
never to be heard from again.

Amen.

5

O heart,
why are you not content?
O spirit,
why are you filled with pride?

For I welcome fear into my home,
I receive it like a friend.
It dwells in my body;
it destroys my peace.

I concern myself with that which is greater than me.
I seek peace and contentment with answers;
I am a fool.

Who was it that spoke life into being?
Who demanded the waters be poured out across the
   earth,
who put a leash on the mountains?
Who controls the temper of the skies,
who causes the rains to fall
and the thunder to shake?
Who separated the East from the West,
the heavens from the earth?
But One.

Only One did,
and He rested on the seventh day.

O soul,
this is your God.
This is your Father,
O broken spirit.
Why do you tremble and shake in a moment of uncertainty,
knowing this is the same God who cares for you?
This same God who walked on water,
who watches and knows your coming and your going.
The same God who overcame life and death
hears and sees your every breath,
knows every hair on your head.

My body is not my refuge,
my spirit is not my strength,
my mind is not my stronghold,
my soul is not my salvation.

My God is.

Amen.

6

My strength is gone.
My faith has withered away,
it has disappeared from the
    surface; I am low.

My eyes sink within me,
I am unrecognizable to those
    who love me.
Look deeply into my eyes,
and you will see a story of
    suffering and misery.
I cannot hide my pain from the
    world,
I cannot escape the hooks of
    destruction.
I am looked upon with pity
    and sorrow,
a life of joy has abandoned me.

I know pain better than I know
    myself,
I see death more than I see life.
Where is my help?
Where does my truth
    come from?
I am torn—

torn between bitterness
    and hope,
suffering and faith,
between what my eyes see and
    what my spirit longs for.
And I have fallen again.
I have given in to deceit;
despair has welcomed me with
    open arms.

When will You come to my
    rescue, O God?
How long will You watch me
    suffer?

I am weak.
In my weakness,
I have turned from the Lord,
for I long to be made whole.
Every moment,
my spirit cries out for rescue.
But the enemy longs to have me,
he attacks me at every turn.

O God, deliver me from the
    jaws of death.

Amen.

7

I have felt the frozen embrace of pain,
the icy breath of death has sent chills down my spine.
The voice of evil has caused my spirit to shake,
I have been enveloped by the cover of darkness.
Fear has rocked me to my core,
anxiety has gripped me with its lifeless embrace of lies.

But here I stand.

My body and spirit stand covered by the marks of war;
my mind is littered with the remains of battle.
With each step,
my bones cry out within me—
even my healing is pain.
Control is my rival;
pride is my downfall.

But mercy is my lifeline.
The sovereignty of One far bigger than me,
providence of He who stands outside of time.
Power that sends the spirit of death away,
like a dog with its tail between its legs.
Such is the status of a Savior,
the rank of a King—

one who melts the frozen embrace of pain,
who commands death away with a word.
He who uses evil for good,
and speaks light that overwhelms darkness in an instant.
The only fear that exists is the fear of the Lord,
who carries all burdens and anxieties.
For His yoke is easy,
and His burden is light.

In my lifelessness,
I am raised up.
In the face of death,
I am upheld.
I cannot be overcome,
for the Lord of all is my commander.

Amen.

8

Where is there an ounce of purity among our people?
Where, I ask, is there a fraction of truth in this place?

In the midst of this culture,
within the wealthiest of times,
I see not a single soul of peace.
The house of the Lord is swallowed by corruption,
its walls are painted with evil.
Outside its doors,
the world is burning—
burning in a pit of frail identity.
The people stumble across the lands,
eyes seeking everything but others.

The pursuit of self commands every eye—
not a single one sees the truth.
Entitlement wreaks havoc on our brothers,
pride blocks the minds of our sisters;
we are wholly unwhole.
The enemy makes his stronghold in our selfish nature,
he burrows into layers of self-righteousness.
No one is free from his elusive sociopathy,
causing hate to boil deep within us.

Who among us is free?
Is there just one with a pure heart?
I see not a single one outside my window,
I see not a single one in the mirror.
For I lead the broken,
I am first in the line of evil.
I do not see an ounce of goodness in me,
I lack a single breath of righteousness.

How, Lord,
can You look upon this earth?
O Father,
have mercy on us!
Undeservedly, You have rescued my spirit;
abundantly, You have delivered my soul.
Yet still, I seek the things of this world,
weightless treasures consume my mind.
I will turn from my foolish ways;
redemption is my only hope.

O my God, cause Your children to rise again!
As the world spins,
so Your will must be done.

The body of Christ is crying out for truth;
your people are drowning in self-reliance,
O, how we need a Savior!

Cause us to turn from evil,
to abandon our wicked nature
until the day of Your return.
Empower Your chosen sons,
equip Your chosen daughters.
Let us rescue this world of comfortable death!

Arise, O saints,
come forward with boldness!
The God of Creation beckons—
answer His call!

Amen.

9

I have no peace in this life
apart from You, O God.
There is no joy in my presence
when I turn my back on You.
I am lost and empty,
foolishly critical and baselessly bitter,
when I walk without Your Spirit.
Why, O spirit of mine,
do you depart from your Maker?

I cannot,
I will not,
live this way.
For when I am without You,
I am utterly without purpose.

Therefore, I confess my iniquities;
they are too many to count.
I submit to You my burdens;
they are too heavy to carry.
Restlessly, I lay down my brokenness;
I am a child of weakness.
O, the joy that comes with knowing the Creator!
How vast His mercies are upon me!
For I am wholly undeserving,
yet You give me power when You forgive.

No longer will I abuse Your grace;
I will not belittle my transgressions.
Instead, I will walk with my eyes fixed on You,
I will condemn the sin that rots my body and mind.
There is power in Your grace,
courage in Your love;
I am a fool to take advantage of Your justice.
Remove the blindness from my eyes,
destroy the deception in my mind.
Root out the temptation in my heart,
instill the truth in my hands.
For I am not a being who must give in to sin;
I am a child who can choose the way of life.

Hold me tight, O Father,
do not let me disappear from Your gaze.
Take hold of my life,
put justice in my heart.
For where Your Spirit resides,
no evil can take hold.

I will walk in the power of truth,
I will stand firm in the presence of temptation.
For You have not given me a spirit of timidity,
but one of power, love, and self-discipline.

Amen.

10

Pride seeks to devour me.
From the moment I rise in the morning,
until I lay my head to rest at night,
selfishness pursues me.

Depart from me,
evil pride!
Be gone from before me,
chaotic self-centeredness!

I am like an addict,
a starving animal,
one who cannot stop prioritizing myself.
What is the remedy for my addiction?
Is there a prescription for this illness?

The world reinforces this notion,
culture celebrates this sickness.
Yet inside of me,
there is war.
Within my heart,
I cannot justify myself as enough.
For I know better than anyone
just how incapable
unable
self-serving
unsteady
broken
I am.

Listen to my words, brothers and sisters,
hear my cry!
The foundation for a life worth living
is the abandonment of yourself.
The remedy for your brokenness
is to love others first.

You cannot sustain yourself;
others will surely let you down.

There is One who will always provide—
He who has never failed—
a King worth loving,
a God worth serving.
And what, you ask,
did He do?

He did no wrong,
and laid down His life for you.

Amen.

11

My legs are heavy,
my mind is weak.
I cannot find any comfort,
I do not know freedom.
Pain is my anger,
trauma is my bitterness,
pride is my rage.

I am tense.
Overflowing with fire,
I cannot understand this life.
I do not understand my suffering;
it is a mysterious beast.
I cannot comprehend my afflictions,
they tear me apart.
When I am alone,
evil crawls toward me;
it sucks me in.
I give in to the darkness.
I rest with my sorrows.
I lose hope.

I do not see any justice.
Why is this burden upon me?
I have been told of the Creator,
yet this burden remains.
Surely a loving God would heal!
He would lift me out of my misery,
He would destroy my enemies.

I am cursed by pride,
I am infected with foolishness,
I do not know truth.

Who am I?
A liar
a cheater
a thief
a selfish human.

Yet when Christ saw no justice,
full of burden on the cross,
He called out to this same loving Father . . .
but the nails remained.
His misery became my forgiveness;
His burden became my freedom;
His destruction became my justification.
Therefore, I say to darkness,

"I choose life,
for my God, in death,
chose me."

Amen.

12

Beckon me to walk in faith,
O Lord.
For I am weak,
but You, my God,
You are strong.
Be my refuge and my strength,
for I am ill with sin.

Comfort me, O Father,
restore strength to my bones,
for I am paralyzed,
consumed by fear,
afraid to walk.
So I will run to You,
I will take shelter in
    Your arms.

Strengthen me, O mighty
    Creator,
give me endurance.
I am not made for the
    shadows,
not created for false comforts.
You made me with power.
You breathed life into my
    lungs;
I was not born to be weak.

You are my Daily Bread,
my Source,
my King,
my Savior.

And You, O God,
cannot lose.
Lift me up,
give me faith,
I will live.
Destroy my fear,
conquer my enemies,
I will serve Your name.

Blessed be our God.
Blessed are His children.
Restore our faith.

Amen.

13

I am confronted by that which I ignored:

my vast limitations,
waves of inability.
Anger ensues, bitterness boils,
I am overcome with sadness.

O Father,
You feel impossible
when sickness surrounds me.
You feel distant
as suffering suffocates me.
What can I do?
I can rely on others,
on myself, or on You.

I know You are the right answer, O God,
but I am stubborn,
and I wonder why You will not rescue me.

What must it be like,
dwelling on high?

Seeing that Your very creation,
that which You sent Your Son to die for,
raises a fist to You,
condemning Your ways,
cursing Your name,
lacking in faith.

All of these things and more
I do, and I am.

As condemnation settles in my heart,
I choose it.
As curses form on my lips,
I send them forth like arrows.
As faith leaves my soul,
I do not resist.

Forgive me, forgive me, O Lord.
I am defeated by life,
exhausted by living,
broken by evil.

I am desperate for You—
for Your power, Your presence,
for Your mercy, Your forgiveness.
I am desperate, more than I know.

Come, Father, please.

I cannot sink into death once more.
Please come.

Amen.

PART 2

FROM

DESPAIR

TO LAMENT

We . . .
are overcome with emotion
don't know how to feel
can't process what is happening
which leads to . . .
despair.

In my distress I called to the LORD;
I called out to my God. From His
temple He heard my voice; my cry
came to His ears.
(2 Samuel 22:7)

He . . .
who hears our distress
who knows the depths of emotion
who wept over His best friend
calls us into . . .
His unwavering commitment to listen.

14

Father,
keep my feet from stumbling,
for my legs wobble and my feet are weary.
Hold me upright with Your strong right hand;
do not let Your presence be far from me.
O Father, be near,
bring Your truth in closer.

My body cries out for mercy,
with each passing day it builds anger
    against me.

My soul shouts for strength,
with each passing day it longs for the river of
    truth.

Do not cause me to fall, O Lord,
strengthen me through the redemption of the
    Cross.
Uphold my broken bones,
tie down my spirit with Your mercy.
For without You my eyes would shut,
never to open again.
But with You,
my joy is set before me.
For as long as I have breath,
I will praise Your name and carry on.

Let my words be a sweet sound in the heavens;
may my actions be a beautiful aroma in the courts.
Wash my heart with the blood of the Lamb,
and purify me according to Your forgiveness.
Equip my hands,
that they might bless the Kingdom until my last day.

Deliver me, Father, rescue me,
so that I might praise Your name forever.

Amen.

15

Night and day,
I call out to you.
Morning and evening,
I cry out in desperation for healing.

I demand,
I desire,
I beg
that this pain would pass,
that this trauma would subside,
that release would finally reign,
that this body,
mind,
and spirit would be restored,
and that my Father would ordain the work of
     my hands.

Should I go on like this,
or no longer beg for healing?
Should I shut my mouth and carry on,
or cry out for healing until that moment comes?

For I am lost,
unsure how to move forward or break free.

Father,
come and rescue me.
Hear my insistent cries and act with grace.
For if my only hope were justice,
my only opportunity righteousness,
I would fall short,
never to rise again.

Yet I have hope in Jesus,
the Son of Man.
It is through Him that I call out for healing,
for rebirth and restoration,
for the sake of the Kingdom alone.

Not my will ever, Father,
but Yours always be done.

Amen.

16

I am downcast
empty
distraught.
This suffering follows me;
dark clouds consume all of my days.

Father, I submit now,
because I have no other option.
You have blessed me so deeply,
but right now,
all I feel is hurt.

At Your feet
I lay my spirit.
Broken and weak,
I fall before the throne of my Savior.
How long can I suffer, Lord?
When will this pain be removed from me?
Come now,
do not wait any longer,
for my hope blows away with the wind;
clarity hides itself from me.

My days have been filled with anguish.
I look behind me,
and all I see is trouble;
I look ahead and see despair waiting.
Heal me now, O Lord,
take this cup away from me,
for I cannot bear it.
Bring a massacre on the evil that surrounds me;
destroy it with Your right hand in an instant.

I am on my knees.
I cannot bear to lift my head.
Go forth before me,
clear a path ahead of me,
and I will rejoice at Your name.
I will sing praise with every breath;
my hands will serve Your kingdom.
In your mercy, Father,
save me.

Declare victory for your child;
let your name be conqueror in this place.

Amen.

17

Father, my soul cries out in desperation,
my spirit shatters in despair,
when I consider separation from Your mercy.
For if I knew not of your grace,
I would no longer wish to live.
I would give myself over to dust and ashes,
never to be heard from again.
The pain would be too great;
destruction would have its way with me.

But . . .
You, O Lord,
pull me from the ashes.
You pick me up from the pit of despair.
You hold me close.
With a voice like thunder, You say:

Beloved, come and rise again,
the depths of My mercy will set you free.
As far as the East is from the West,
so have your sins been separated from you.
Listen to My voice;
hear My call.
You have been sanctified by the blood of the Lamb.
In your depravity, your desolation,
you have continued to seek your Holy Creator.

Be set free,
for My righteousness has covered the costs.
You will see My goodness.
My mercy will walk beside you.
Nothing will stand between us again—
this I promise.

I will worship the King forevermore.
His goodness brings tears to my eyes,
and trembling to my knees.
I will never seek my identity elsewhere again,
for You are my only hope.

Amen.

18

What have you allowed upon me, O Lord?
Why do you see to my destruction?
When will I know freedom,
and will I ever see these shackles broken?

I must ask,
for my light has been removed from me,
my cup is empty.
You watch me as I stumble through each day,
as I fall weak with every passing moment.
My strength is gone;
it left me long ago.
Where can I go from here?
Downward I fall
to new depths of suffering.

My life has gone from me;
in its place death and deceit fill my spirit.
I know nothing of happiness;
rest left me in a heap of ashes.
My soul aches—
I long for it all to end.

You, God, strike down the wicked;
You destroy the arrogant.
When You look upon me,
is this what You see?

For I look at my neighbor,
I see evil and destruction around every corner.
Yet You uphold their lives,
their cups overflow,
happiness is their welcome companion.

But me?
I spend my moments with death on my doorstep.
Discomfort fills my lungs,
pain sinks its teeth into my body.
I cannot escape.

In a moment,
You could look upon me with grace,
and it would be over.
But this is not my reality;
healing is a stranger I do not know.
Strike me down, Father,
if Your will is to see my end.
Or lift me up from the presence of death,
if You will to see me live.

I will praise Your name
no matter what.

Amen.

19

Another morning has come,
and with it I have broken down.
My body has corrupted me,
my mind has stolen control of my being.
I am overcome, overwhelmed,
because I find no rest.
Fear has demanded my attention,
anxiety cripples the depths of my soul—
I cannot breathe.

Father, I have lost everything,
for I have now lost myself.
I am surrounded by evil;
the enemy crouches around every corner.
He attacks me mercilessly—
I cannot see.

O my soul,
will you stand idly by?
Frail mind of mine,
have you no fight?
The prince of this earth takes only what he is given;
the God of the universe does as He chooses;
and yet you, O soul, have given in to this enemy.
The Father of all truth knocks at the door of your heart,
yet you stand motionless,
refusing to let Him in.

Where is your victory, O my spirit?
In a moment,
you are tossed by the wind,
dragged by the waters of the current.
The Lord your God has stretched out His mighty hand,
yet you drift by,
consumed by the enemy's lies.
Have you no backbone?
Will you continue allowing evil to sit at your table?
Or will you feast at the table of the Lord your God,
where there is strength forevermore,
where your cup will overflow?

You are on the path to death,
frail body of mine.
You are leaping into the mouth of the devil,
anxious spirit of mine.
Turn away now;
take hold of the rock of salvation.

Amen.

20

Who is this God?
When you speak of His strength,
do you mean it?
When you consider His power,
do you believe it?
For we have read about it for generations;
we have filled pages with words declaring it.
Yet it has lost its meaning;
its magnitude has become watered down.
We are sheep,
foolish and brash,
surrounded by comfort and distraction.
We do not know this God;
our words are distant from our hearts.

O my soul,
you are a fool.
Feeble mind of mine,
you know but a shadow of this God.

My God and my Father,
wake me out of this ignorant slumber!
O Creator and King,
take hold of my spirit,
grip my soul!
Forgive me for my shallow incompetence.
The greatest weapon of evil is dull distraction and comfort.

I am deaf to the sound of Your great Word,
my eyes are blind to the majesty,
the splendor, of my God.
My soul is numb to the power,
the magnificence, of my Savior.
I am a fool, a sinful child.

Jesus Christ, my Lord,
beckon me into Your presence.
Reach down from the heavens,
replace my fear of this world
with the fear of the Lord.
For this world crumbles and falls,
in a moment it could be no more.
But the Word of the Lord has stood for ages;
it has passed down from generation to generation.
Men and women have come and gone;
they are alive in a moment,
in the next, they are nothing.

Yet, Your Word stands.

Therefore, I will trust in You.
For faith elsewhere will surely disappear with the rest.
Awaken my soul,
let me sleep not a moment longer!

Amen.

21

Father, I fall to my knees in
    sorrow,
for my bones cannot hold
    me up.
In my weakness,
I have succumbed to the snare
    of the enemy.
My heart is filled with
    remorse,
my head is full of anguish,
for I am a victim of my selfish
    desires.

Clouds form overhead,
numbness takes hold of
    my body,
I am utterly filled with regret.
The greatest lie of the enemy
is that my actions can do
    no harm.
Yet, O God,
even a moment of foolishness
has my soul burning with fire.

On my left,
guilt seeks my attention.
To my right,
shame invites me to dwell.
Ever at my back is
    exploitation.
My body is covered by scars of
    abuse,
my spirit remembers each
    twisted moment of pain.
The prince of darkness has cut
    me open;
You, O God, lay me bare at
    Your feet.
In self-disgust,
I seek to cover my fractured
    frame.
What have I become?
Blemished
unfit
unclean
disposed of
used
broken.

Yet
Your hand stretches
    toward me,
Your light extends past the
    darkness in my midst.
The body of Christ,
that which was once blemished
unfit
unclean
disposed of
used
broken
stands washed clean.

Forgive my sinful nature,
    my God.
I cannot bear to stand on
    my own,
even a moment longer.
I no longer wish to serve
    myself;
I will be buried in the earth,
unless it is You who lives
    in me.

I cannot stand my own
    reflection,
so I will spend my days gazing
    upon the Father.
Wash me clean, O Lord,
wash over me with the blood
    of the Lamb.

Today is the day I have been
    crucified at last.

Amen.

22

I cannot undo what was done,
I cannot erase what I know.
As my past seeks to devour me,
the present fails to exist.

My body wears the scars of the past—
each one confronts me as I rise in the morning.

But when I am with You,
the storms cannot drown me.
With You beside me,
my soul has peace.

I have never known love like this;
I will never know love any better.
I have never seen mercy like this;
I will never see mercy any better.

You have not changed, O Lord.
You pursued me when I ran,
You were present when I turned my back.
When I cursed You, hated You,
You waited for me.
When the world gave up on me,
You held me close.
This love is indescribable.

Amen.

23

Pick me up out of misery,
bring me out of despair.
Set my gaze upon You,
my feet on solid ground.

You cannot be defeated;
I will be victorious.

Show me the way, O God,
I will go.
Cause me to act, O God,
I will be fearless.

You are a lamp for my feet,
a light for my path.
I cannot bear to be apart
   from You.

My legs are too faint to move;
make me walk.
My mind is too burdened;
force me to go.
My spirit is broken to pieces;
fill me with Your presence.

I am not my own,
I am Yours.

Rid me of my pride,
strip away my fear.
Extinguish my judgment,
destroy my self-reliance.

I do not belong to the world.
I belong to Your kingdom.

You are my strength,
You are my hope.
Make me a new creation,
a child of power,
a child of endurance.

I cannot be overcome,
I am a child of God.
What the enemy intended
   for harm,
God means for good.
Therefore, I will remain
   in Him,
with He who is holy.
I declare the name of the Lord,
there is none greater;
praise His name.

Amen.

PART 3

FROM DEFIANCE TO SUBMISSION

We . . .
don't understand the why
can't understand the how
are overcome by the what
which leads to . . .
defiance.

The LORD thundered from heaven; the
voice of the Most High resounded.
(2 Samuel 22:14)

He . . .
who is slow to anger
who sees the why
who knows the how
calls us into . . .
submission to His will.

24

Why is it
that I have been utterly broken into pieces,
yet I am still not free?

I ignore the mistakes I continue to make,
sins that still grip me,
and place strongholds on my thoughts.
I see now
that my sin,
my shortcomings,
cripple me.
I cannot break free,
because I am not free—

free of myself,
free of my wrongdoing,
free of my fear,
free of my anxieties,
free of my pride—
I am not.

I see the very thing that I ask for,
that I demand,
is the very thing I refuse to rid myself of—me.
How will I have freedom
if I am not free of myself?

How can I have victory
if I am swallowed up by my sinful pride?
For I know that rejoicing comes in the morning,
yet I continue to weep through the night.

I demand the face and presence of my God,
yet I hide in the shadows of my sin.

I will be broken until I am free of myself.
Father, break me until this work of Yours is complete.
And when that day comes,
be merciful to me.
Turn my crying into dancing,
my weeping into rejoicing.

My heart will sing Your praises.
I will not be silent,
for the Lord God will set me free.

Amen.

25

In my impatience,
I speak with rash haste.
In my bitterness,
I speak with words that cut through the air,
piercing the heart of those who listen.
In my ignorance,
I speak with unfounded righteousness,
for I know nothing.
In my foolishness,
my actions flare into a tantrum.

But . . .
patiently, my God waits.
He remains,
bearing the brunt of my attacks;
they fall at his feet as if they were nothing.
My Father lets out a soft smile
as I clench my fists and beat the ground.
He lets my temper tire itself out,
then scoops up my frail body into His hands.
With eyes as deep as the ocean,
and a voice like soft thunder,
He says,

My child, your time will come.
I will not take you past the point you cannot bear.
Your spirit is Mine,
so, too, your body and the complexities within.

I know your scars,
I see the hurt that covers you from head to toe.
Your pain is My pain,
your suffering belongs to Me.
I own your deepest afflictions,
I bear your heaviest burdens,
I know every moment of loneliness.
Not a drop of it has fallen
unknown to Me.

You will know freedom,
your victory will be a song of triumph in the heavenly courts.
You will know My complete goodness
because you have felt the depths of suffering.
You will hear My voice
because you have known the darkness of silence.
You will know the depths of peace
because you have lived the chaos of separation.
You will know genuine love
because you have experienced the lies of temporary pleasures.
You will live a life of empathy
because you have felt the weight of despair.

You will know the perfection of My mercy
because you have lived the depravity of sin.

Amen.

26

My God,
where can I find You?
I know nothing but emptiness and desolation.
My suffering has no end.

Is this the life promised to me?
Day after day,
moment by moment,
my life deteriorates in front of me.
I am haunted by my past.
My future is covered in dark clouds,
my present is painted by pain.

Freedom is far from me,
comfort has abandoned my soul.
Fear and anxiety grip me,
I cannot find an escape.
Some look on me with pity,
others look down on me with judgment.
They know nothing of the destruction that has seized me,
the loss that has rampaged every ounce of my body.

But my peace cannot be found in the heart of humanity,
my comfort is not hidden in the mind of another.
The only contentment I will ever know
is that which I will find in You.

And so I call,
with each burdensome breath I have,
I cry out to my Father.

Come quick,
for I am losing myself.
Evil surrounds me,
the night covers me—I cannot see.
Darkness descends upon me,
I am crippled by pain and shackles of suffering.

I cry to the Lord for help,
for I know He answers His children.

Come quick, Father,
that I may praise Your name everlasting,
for You will bring the victory.

Amen.

27

Am I a fool for questioning?
Am I a child for turning away?
In my exhaustion,
I grow sick of hearing,
"Just a little while longer."
I want answers.
I desire to be whole again.
The depths of my worn spirit cry out.
Does my call for help reach the ears of heaven?
My pride tells me no.

Constantly under attack,
I grow weaker with each passing day.
My enemies feel joy
as they watch me be stripped of my humanity.
How I long to be born again,
a new body, mind, and spirit.
As I look upon the face of death,
I feel an unexpected response:
indifference and numbness.

What have I become?

There exists no worse emotion in the face of death
than indifference.

Too exhausted to continue living,
too indifferent for death,
my spirit is gray.
I am lukewarm,
a bitter taste that hits the tongue.
One looked upon with pity,
yet too dull for association,
my presence is a sour one.
Why do I continue this way?
I have turned my back on the Lord,
yet He gives me breath in the morning.
I curse my God with bitterness,
yet He welcomes me back home with open arms.
I grow numb with indifference at my Father,
yet He sees the beauty in my soul.

Why is this a God I would refuse?

Amen.

Cold
lost
empty
filled with rage,
I am without You.

I cannot contain my bitterness;
self-entitlement rules my head.
Emptiness becomes my only understanding;
I am brought so low that I am paralyzed.
Anxiety grips and shakes me;
the enemy sinks into my core
when I depart from You.

Depression knows my face;
sadness welcomes me in.
Pride licks its lips when I descend near to it;
anger smiles as I boil within.
I am unstable
heartless
meaningless
dead,
I am without You.

O Father,
pull me close to You.
I am crying out for Your love.
I am empty without Your touch.

I cannot walk another step,
I cannot take another breath
if I am without You.
Yet with You I am full,
by Your side I have comfort.
At Your feet I am content,
in Your presence I am home.
Why would I ever stray from You?

I refuse to accept forgiveness;
the enemy weighs too heavily on my heart.
Because I am full of pride,
I cannot see past my flaws.
I am blinded by self-seeking righteousness,
for I cannot accept pure forgiveness.
I do not stand before the Lord with any joy,
only self-contempt and unworthiness.

This keeps me from You;
it causes me to stumble.
Hatred boils within me;
I despise the reflection in the mirror.

How could You forgive this wretch, O Lord?
Though I do not deserve it,
I accept it with rejoicing.

Amen.

29

Father, forgive me.
For I have forgotten Your
  majesty,
I have simplified Your wonder.

Your power has become dull to
  my senses;
Your creation has lost its beauty.
I am like a fool who covers
  his eyes,
one who is oblivious to all
  things.

The Creator of the world
is basic in my eyes.
The God of the oceans and
  seas, moon and stars
is an inconvenience to me.
O, what a wretched fool I am!

King of kings,
Lord of lords,
You made all things.

You spoke,
and the world was;
light burst forth with a word.

The mountains demand
  our gaze,
the skies reflect Your goodness.
The oceans reveal Your depth,
the galaxies declare Your
  magnitude.
I am a fool!
Blind
illiterate
asleep
numb to Your great name.

Praise Your name, O God,
You deserve all praise.
I will humble myself in Your
  presence,
for I cannot bear Your power.
Teach me to remember who
  You are;
I am so quick to forget.

You are God—
Creator
Maker
God.

Amen.

30

Where is Your justice, O God?
Where is my peace?

Time and time again,
I watch evil stand victorious.
I watch the criminal walk free.
He smiles at me without guilt.
A man of corruption,
one without any shame,
gets to carry on.

And what of me?

My eyes are filled with tears,
my body is ash and rubble,
I feel no hope.
I bear the bruises of deep hurt;
scars cover me inside and out.
Fire rages within me,
darkness washes over me like water.
I cannot stand this injustice,
it eats away at my soul;
I have no peace.

Is this my life?

Where is my bounty, O Father? Where is my victory?
I am empty.

O, My child,
I am with you.
I am justice,
I am peace.
I am your bounty,
I am the victory.

Draw near to Me, My child,
You are My beloved treasure.
Do not depart from Me,
for I am making you new.
I will not leave you,
nor forsake you.
I am your God.

I cannot be overcome,
justice will prevail.
Your story will be told,
you are set free.

Go forth, do not wait.
Be a beacon of hope, a light in darkness.
Do not fear, do not worry,
the Lord your God is with you.

Amen.

31

My tongue is a weapon,
harsh and biting.
It manipulates, curses,
sets my body on fire.
The tongue is a spark,
which fills me with rage;
I am unclean.

Teach me to speak with grace.
Create in me a selfless mind,
that which leads to words
    of love.
For I am quick to speak,
and slow to listen.

My words are a thorn in my
    flesh;
my lips bring poison upon me.

Forgive me, O Lord,
for my wicked haste.
How quickly I condemn
    others,
how slowly I judge myself;
I am blind.
Curse my tongue,
which causes me to sin.

Bring newness upon me,
    O God,
gentleness upon my lips.
Give me patience, not envy;
give me humility,
not bitterness.
Cause Your Word to be
    my own,
that I may speak with truth.
I must treasure Your thoughts,
Your commands,
Your Spirit,
that I may gain Christ.

You are patient,
You are steadfast,
You are pure.

You are just,
You are righteous,
You are holy.

Help me not to forget.

Amen.

PART 4

FROM
GRIEF TO
RESCUE

We . . .
grow exhausted with emotion
see the failures of our reactions
feel the same way we felt before
which leads to . . .
grief.

He reached down from on high and took
hold of me; He drew me out of deep waters.
(2 Samuel 22:17)

He . . .
who sees us as His beloved
who never sleeps nor slumbers
who holds the earth in His palm
calls us into . . .
His eagerness to rescue us.

32

Father,
I am exhausted.
I am wrong.
I am fed up.
I am weak.

I am weary.
I am not able.
I am human.
I am sinful.

Be my breath.
Be my light.
Be my truth.
Be my strength.
Be my redemption.
Be my forgiveness.
Be my everything.

I am wholly Yours;
not a single breath is my own.
Give me more of You always,
and less of me forevermore,
that I might never stray from You.

Amen.

33

I am just a human
infant
child.
Hopeless on my own,
I wander through each day.
My enemy presses in,
he steals my breath and I become weak.
My body trembles,
my bones shake;
there is a war going on and it cannot
    be seen.
Affliction has taken its stranglehold,
pain has become my closest friend.
My body fails to recognize me,
my mind turns on itself.

What was once most natural is now my
    biggest hurdle;
what I once knew is a distant memory.
Where did I go so wrong
that I have ended up here?
Here, where I sit and do not move.
Here, where I spend my days wasting away.

If these walls could talk,
they would join me with tears.
They would look at me with pity.
They would see me and say,
"There lies the shadow of a human,
one who lived not knowing he had everything."

What I once had,
I will never have again.
Yet I would lose it all twice over
if it meant my Savior would find me.

For in this place He found me—
not when I had everything,
but when I had nothing.

For if in my nothingness
I gain my Savior,
then I have all that I need.

Amen.

3 4

Long are the nights I have spent
tossing and turning,
eyes heavy but still wide awake.
Long are the days I have spent
stumbling and seething.

Anxiety and bitterness surround me;
I cry out to You, O God,
my hands tremble as I reach for a lifeline.
Do not be blind,
do not turn away;
cherish me as Your child.
Restore me with Your waves of mercy.

Long have I suffered,
but long will be the days
that the face of the Lord
will shine upon me.
From the depths,
He will restore me.
From the darkness,
He will call me forth to light.
I will shout for joy,
I will sing Your praise.

Your people will know the goodness and
    favor of the Lord,
for those who live by righteousness.

For what good are blessings,
without the ability to share with another?
What good is life,
without hope in restoration?

For these things I cry out, Father,
my soul longs for them alone—
a soul that can reflect this new spirit,
a community that is rooted in our Heavenly
    Father,
and the opportunity to serve Your kingdom
for the rest of my days.

Amen.

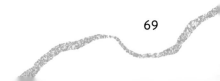

35

I long to be made whole again.
From the moment I rise,
until I close my eyes in the evening,
every piece of me longs to be made complete.
My body aches,
it groans for healing.
My mind finds no rest,
it cries out for comfort.
My soul is depleted,
it thirsts for peace.

I long to be made whole,
though I realize I will not find it in this life.
My body aches
for that which cannot be found.
My mind seeks
for that which is impossible.
My soul thirsts
for that which will never come.
For I realize I am a foreigner in this world,
a traveler who does not belong—
an imperfect child,
who seeks wholeness from an imperfect world.

Yet, in all of this,
I see everything I long for:
a perfect God seeking a wholly imperfect child.

In this notion alone,
my body can find healing,
my mind can find a glimmer of comfort,
and my soul can find a fullness of hope.

Though I know that in this life
I will never be fully complete,
I see more clearly than ever
that eternity with my God is the only option.

Amen.

36

O my soul,
when was the last time you knew comfort?
O spirit,
when did you last rest?
O fleeting mind,
have you ever known peace?
Body of mine,
when were you last content?

For I feel the heat of battle,
but I do not take up any armor.
I see evil as it descends upon me,
yet I do not hold firm.
I put my faith in flesh and blood,
but flesh and blood know me not.

How do I claim to believe in this God
when I refuse to lay my anxiety to rest?
I do not know this God of peace,
if my moments are consumed by fear.

How is this body a temple of the Holy Spirit
when my mind refuses to let it be my strength?
I do not know this Spirit of truth,
if my days are filled with trembling and confusion.

How is my soul covered by the blood of Jesus
when I refuse to trust the promises He has given?
I do not know this Son of Man,
if I do not accept His words of truth.

Humbly and meekly,
I crawl back to the foot of the throne.
I do not have the strength to lift my head,
but my soul longs to remain in Your presence.
I cannot be moved from this place;
surely my life would wither away.

Then Your hand reached out to me,
You lifted my head.
In Your eyes,
I saw my eternity.

All that I carried melted away.

Amen.

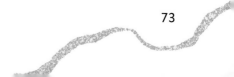

37

I have explored every avenue.
I have walked through paths of darkness.
I have been a prisoner to myself,
an inmate shackled by the chains of my suffering.
I have been subdued by evil.
I have known the scent of the enemy.
Destruction has been a close companion of mine,
pain closer than a friend.
I have felt the degrading hands of abuse;
my skin has been pierced by the onslaught of hurt.

Yet, I have a God who loves me.
My Maker cares for me,
my Father knows me.
My God does not just see my pain,
He feels it and knows it.
My Redeemer does not ignore my suffering;
He delivers me according to His perfect understanding.

In my stubbornness,
I condemn what He has put me through.
In my bitterness,
I demand He answer me according to my terms.
All the while I forget:
He is God and I am not.

He does not diminish my pain,
nor does He abandon my reality.
Rather,
He gives me the means to press on,
a desire to pursue eternal truth—
peace that transcends circumstances,
wisdom that grows with hurt.

For what is knowledge,
if it has not been tested?
What is peace,
if there has been no pain?
What is joy,
if there has been no loss?
Empty
shallow
false.

I refuse to be deceived;
I will put my faith in You.

Amen.

38

O small mind of mine,
you know little,
though you claim to know much.

Father, I lay down all that I have,
I confess all that I lack.
Open and desolate,
the enemy seeks to exploit every gap.
For he can turn nothing into something,
can attack in a moment of weakness.

I am overwhelmed
by that which I cannot control;
I am weak in the midst of intense struggle.
But You raise me up in my longing.
You give me strength when I fail.
You are the God of providence.
Force me to turn from self-reliance,
to tear down the facade of self-entitlement,
so I may look upon Your face.

Creator, You are good;
You will not withhold bountiful mercy.
You are not a God of suppression;
You unleash Your love on Your children.
Surely, if You descended upon this place,
I could not withstand Your majesty.

Woe is me;
I am not fit to live,
but I am certain to die.
In my depravity,
I have grown fearful to live.
I am consumed by my insufficiency,
burdened by the thorns of the enemy.
He has taught me to be uncertain in every moment,
to doubt that which is simple.

Therefore, raise me up again.
In Your goodness,
destroy my enemy.
In Your power,
wipe away the death that entangles me.
In Your mercy,
forgive Your beloved,
for I am a child of foolish brokenness.

One thing I know, O Father,
of which I am certain:
a life of pain and suffering is worth it,
if the Kingdom of God is gained.

Amen.

39

Why is it, O Lord,
that I cannot receive Your grace?
Why is it, O God,
that I cannot accept love from the Father?
In my head,
I am a reject;
in my heart,
I am a waste.
I cannot see past my own insufficiency.

Rather, I dwell with my sin;
it paralyzes my bones.
I take refuge in my brokenness.
I find comfort in self-exploitation.

When I look upon myself,
what do I see?
A victim
a fool
a madman—
too far gone is me.
Forgive me, O Father,
forgive and break me free,
for the enemy exploits me,
he takes hold of me.

I long to be free,
I long to be whole.
Yet, when You offer me forgiveness,
I refuse to accept it.
Is it my pride,
my arrogance,
that blinds my sight?
Is it lack of faith,
lack of trust,
that blocks out Your love?

I cannot speak,
my words will not flow.
My head is in shambles,
my thoughts will not go.
All I know is I am rageful,
I am ready to burst.
I am filled with emptiness,
I am down in the dirt.

Bring me answers, O Lord,
speak truth over me,
for I am so weary,
I am too weary to be.

Amen.

40

When I look in front of me,
I am overcome by my inability and insufficiency.
I cannot see out of the darkness in my environment,
I cannot find any joy in my days.

But when I meditate on the promises of the Lord,
there is a peace that gives me reason.
For when I rise to a new day,
when I understand the promises of faith,
my environment becomes secondary—
a slight affliction,
a moment of pain
in the scope of eternal fullness.

Therefore,
let me confess my utter lack of all things.
Father, continue to humble Your little one,
for I am nothing if not stubborn and forgetful.

I have not known a single soul
who has regretted a life of faith—
is there one?
Yet, I know many who regret a life of empty pursuit.

I will indulge in the life of saints,
to be filled with the power of the Lord.
Those who find peace in every circumstance
triumph in the midst of trial.

Without this, my life would end,
it is so simple.
Therefore,
let me choose faith.

Amen.

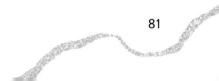

41

Anxious thoughts are my companion;
as I rise,
so, too, does worry.
As I seek,
fear stalks me in every place.
Even as I rest,
anxiety pursues my soul.

O Father,
I am a fool to live like this.
Fear is crippling,
worry destroys my mind,
I cannot carry on this way.
For I know whom I am to fear,
yet I do not.
I choose to fear man,
not the Lord.

Set me free, gracious Judge,
set me free.
For I know
freedom exists in the fear of the Lord.
Give me wisdom, God,
to know this truth.
Break the chains of anxiety,
by making me Your servant.

I refuse to give into this temptation,
I will fight with endurance and strength.
Forgive my foolishness, O Father,
I know so little.
Forgive my self-reliance, O King,
I know that I am weak.

I will not wait idly by,
I will not be a passenger.
I am a conqueror;
I will conquer this sin by Your grace.
You can do all things,
for You are God.
You cannot lose,
for You are I Am.

You will conquer,
You will overcome,
You will have victory
over my affliction.

Amen.

42

I have suffered so long,
it has become normality.
My pain, my afflictions,
are as constant as the sunshine.
Each day that I rise,
I know hurt will rise too.
Each evening as I lay my head down,
burden rests with me.

I struggle to find hope,
as the weight of constant suffering buries me.
My eyes are heavy, my bones are weak;
sickness does not depart from me.

O Lord God, I long for rescue.
O dear Father, I long to be free.
My soul is faint with emptiness,
my mind cannot sustain;
I have such need.
O, how I wish to give in,
to give up and be defeated.
What a joy it would be to my enemies,
they would sing and shout for victory.

So, I carry on today.

My God is not a fool,
my King does not lose.
He cares for His children,
He defeats every opposition.
Whom shall I fear?

The enemy cannot keep me down,
for the Lord cannot be defeated.

My Conqueror and my King,
lift me up!
Bring power to my soul,
endurance to my mind,
forgiveness to my spirit.

You overcome all things.
Hear my cry and rescue me;
let it be done.

I will rest in Your presence,
taking shelter in Your Word.
I will remember how You delivered me,
recalling all that You have done.
I am Your warrior,
Your hands and feet.

You do not lose.

Amen.

43

I cannot run from You,
I cannot hide.
Though I wish to cover my face,
You are with me;
I do not deserve a God like You.

No sooner do I curse Your name
than Your love is poured out
  on me.
No sooner do I criticize Your ways
than Your goodness is revealed
  to me.

I am overcome with emotions,
drowning in tears.
My body is suffering,
my mind is in pain,
my soul is full of sorrow,
life seeks to steal my joy.
How I long to be set free.

I cannot recall a life of freedom,
I do not remember a life without
  affliction;
all that I know is hurt.

Come to my aid,
be my rescue,

for I am weak.
I am brokenhearted,
buried by disappointment;
be near.

Denounce this evil,
deliver me with healing.
I cannot dwell anywhere else
but with You.
Great is Your faithfulness,
righteous are Your ways;
I know nothing of Your
  providence.

For who am I to consider Your
  ways unjust?

Let me put my hope in You.
You will deliver me,
You will set me free,
You will heal me;
You are God.

I will praise Your name,
I will follow Your ways,
I will trust in You;
You are God.

Amen.

PART 5

FROM WANDERING TO OBEDIENCE

We . . .
search for meaning
long for answers
seek different vices
which leads to . . .
wandering.

The LORD has dealt with me according to my
righteousness; according to the cleanness of my hands
he has rewarded me. For I have kept the ways of the
LORD; I am not guilty of turning from my God.
(2 Samuel 22:21–22)

He . . .
who seeks our hearts
who is the source of all meaning
who desires to dwell in us
calls us into . . .
the purpose found in obedience to Him.

44

Lord, how long will You let evil have its way with me?
How long will my prayers go unanswered?
Will I live out the rest of my days in pain and suffering,
until I take my last breath and return to the ground?
Will discomfort be my closest acquaintance?
Will trials of all kinds be my daily bread?
Will I spend my days laboring?
Will my work be in vain?

Two things I ask, Father:
that my labor not be in vain,
and that my suffering not be such that I turn my back on You.
Uphold me until I am delivered from these trials,
so that I might shout for joy for Your great name.
For my days will be filled with worship,
my lips will praise Your power.

Hear my cry, O Lord,
let this day of terror run its course.
Raise me up, according to Your goodness.
Set me free because of Your love.
Restore me through Your miraculous power.

Forever Your name will reign in my spirit.
My lips will shout praise until my body takes its last breath,
for I will know that my tears have not been sown in vain.

Amen.

45

I am fed up, I am done.

Day after day,
moment after moment,
I stand still.
Nothing changes,
nothing loosens,
nothing improves.
And not a moment goes by without pain—
not one.
Not a second goes by without discomfort—
not one.

When will it end?
Why do You lay my head down at night?
Why do You cause me to rise in the morning?

Where is Your healing, miraculous God?
Where is Your comfort, loving Father?
Where is Your deliverance, all-knowing Creator?

I've searched
rested
cried
screamed
hidden
stepped into the open—
yet I cannot find You.

I cannot see Your face.
I cannot hear Your whisper.
I cannot feel Your presence.
Where are You?

How do You look upon me in this moment?
Do You turn Your head in anger,
scoffing in disgust?
Are You cast down in sadness,
or do You not even see?
Do You consider why You ever died
for a wretch like me?

I am out of solutions,
my cup has run dry twice over.
My body shakes,
my feet fall weak beneath me.
I am nothing.

Emptiness and despair are my closest
    companions.

Do You hear me?
Do You know me?
Do You care?

Amen.

46

How can I escape anxiety
when I have nowhere to move?
How will I find rest
when my body conspires against me?
Where is my freedom
when I am trapped and shackled by chains?

My mind has built in me a prison,
my body has attached itself to exhaustion.
I have no hope in anything of myself,
no ability to fix that which is broken.
Pain has frozen me in place,
suffering is all that I know.
Each day passes by with no progress,
I watch the seasons change from my window.
I forget what it's like to move, to live,
to run and jump,
to laugh and sing with joy.

That which I took for granted
is all that I long for—
to feel myself again,
to wake up with expectation and ambition.
How foolish I was
to waste the smallest of things.

Where can I look, O Father?
Have You left me once and for all?
For I am low,
I am drowning.
I no longer wish to carry on in this way,
if this is the way of my life.
Where is my hope?
Where is my healing?
Where is my purpose?

Where are You, my God, where are You?

Amen.

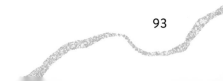

47

When will my time come, O God?
How long must I continue to wait, Father?

Long have I hurt;
I have brought my pain into the light.
I have asked for salvation,
cried out for rescue,
yet all I hear is silence.

Deliver me from the grasp of my enemy;
do not delay any longer,
for I am drowning.
The current has pulled me under;
I cannot breathe.

Drive out this darkness with light;
overcome that which is too great for me.
I am humbled by my own insufficiency.
I have seen the sin of the world;
I have known the deceit of the enemy.

By Your grace,
I am forgiven.
In my pride,
I turn from You,
yet You wait patiently for my return.

You see my iniquities,
You know my brokenness,
yet You welcome me home with open arms.

I know that You will restore me,
for there remains work to be done.
I know that You will strengthen me,
for there is breath still in my lungs.
I know that You will confirm me,
for You have humbled me back to You.
I know that You will establish me,
for You have inclined my heart
to serve Your kingdom forever.

Let it be so.

Amen.

48

In the midst of my struggle I wonder,
Is the hand of the Lord turned against me?
Am I being purged from the outside in?
Am I being laid barren,
with no stone left uncovered?
For every bone,
every muscle,
every ounce of me cries out.
I simply cannot hide from this wave of destruction.

Has the Lord, in His wisdom,
made this body to be cut open?
Are my wounds the work of His judgment?
No.

I am burdened with sin so great that I cannot look
    upon my Lord,
not even for a moment.
Yet, I am His,
and He calls me child, beloved.

Therefore, I know without any doubt,
the enemy desires to exploit my whole soul;
he seeks to devour every ounce of peace.

Yet, here I stand—
Mangled, beaten, unwound, spilled out;
I am completely incomplete.
But my Father has drawn a line in the sand.
He has stood with me in my troubles,
been next to me in the face of death.

And now,
I stand before my Savior,
and He gazes upon me.

I know your pain,
I have been poured out like water.
I know your brokenness,
I have been cut open and beaten.
I know your emptiness,
I have been separated from the Father.
I know your weariness,
I have been too feeble to take a breath.
I know your enemy,
I have overcome him before.
I know you, my child,
I have been with you for eternity.

Just as I have overcome,
so shall you.
Just as I have conquered,
so shall you.
Just as I have forgiven,
so shall you.
Just as I have lived,
so shall I live in you.

You lift up my head,
Your glory is blinding.

I am a conqueror and coheir with Christ.

Amen.

49

God of all gods,
Lord of all lords,
who can compare to You?

From days of old,
You have not changed.
Your words remain,
Your power is present,
there are none like You.
When I consider Your magnitude,
as I watch the world spin,
I can't help but feel unworthy.

I struggle for purpose,
I worry about meaning.
My pursuits turn to dead ends,
my desires wither without water.
I fail to understand
that my ultimate longing for this life
    brings emptiness.

Rather, I will rise with the morning,
and put my trust in You.
I will seek Your kingdom,
Your truth.
I will walk with the legs You gave me;
I will pursue Your Word.

For if Your will be done,
how will anything stand in the way?

Raise me out of this fog, O Lord,
lift me up on Your powerful wings.
Set my feet on solid ground.
I will pursue the will You have for me.
I refuse to sit back,
I will not waste,
I will go.

Amen.

50

Speak to me, O God;
lead me in Your ways, Father.
Do not let me grow complacent,
for You are far too able.
Reinforce my faith in You,
for I am anxious about all things.

Keep me from wandering;
incline my spirit to action.
You did not waste a thing
when You created me,
Your child.
Do not let me be deceived by dead ends;
lead me to seek You even in
    hopelessness.

For You are boundless;
Your power cannot be contained.

If You walk before me,
I will not be beaten.
If You walk beside me,
I cannot fall.
If You walk behind me,
I will never perish.

In the monotony of confusion,
show me Your wild creativity.
In the weariness of my empty pursuits,
open my eyes to Your work.

I will remember that which You
    have done;
I will press on.
If Your plans are to prosper me,
I am a fool to give up.

You are the God who spoke a word
and unleashed blinding light throughout
    the earth.
That same power exists in me.
For as the Spirit hovered over the waters,
He makes a temple out of me.

Why, then, would I ever give up?
Why would I ever give in?
I will not.
Your ways will not be thwarted.
Your power cannot be challenged.
You will reign.

Amen.

PART 6

FROM

CROSSROADS

TO JUSTICE

We . . .
hit rock bottom
can't see a way out
have no other place to turn
which leads to . . .
a crossroad between life and death.

To the faithful you show yourself faithful, to the
blameless you show yourself blameless. . . . You, LORD,
are my lamp; the LORD turns my darkness into light.
(2 Samuel 22:26, 29)

He . . .
who suffered beyond all suffering
who sent His Son to die on the cross
who bore all sin though He knew no sin
calls us into . . .
the perfect balance of His justice.

53

For your name's sake, O Lord,
make me well.
Forgive me;
bless my hands and the actions that flow
  from them.
Heal my brokenness,
restore me and build me up again.

According to Your great love,
keep my ways pure and holy.
Wipe my record clean;
instill goodness in me, Your child,
and make my paths clear.
Bring me into Your Holy Temple at heaven's gates,
let me dwell there forever.

For I am nothing if not Yours,
and I am hopeless without Your perfect love.

Take my life away,
but do not take Yourself away from me.

Amen.

54

I have choices:
gratitude or pride,
purity or sin,
life or death.

I will fight the good fight;
I will not give into myself easily.
There is a war that exists.
It is not flesh and blood;
it is rooted deeply in the spiritual.

Therefore, I will fight—
fight to defeat my own mindset,
my own negative thoughts,
for that way lies destruction.
Through the grace of the Spirit,
I can control how I think,
I can control how I respond,
I can control how I react.
Therefore, I will.

The Lord has given me the mind of Christ,
His Holy Spirit makes a home in me.
I cannot do this on my own,
but I can and will through the grace of the Spirit.

Amen.

55

If you, O Lord, wished to strike me down,
it would be done.
Nothing would remain, no piece of me;
the memory of my life would be gone in a moment.
Therefore, I know
the Lord has promised me a future—

one of joy,
one of peace and love,
one of depth and hurt,
one of impact and faith.
For I know my God.
He has set my feet on trembling ground,
so that my spirit would be humbled.

I hear a voice say,
This, too, shall pass.

Just a little while longer,
until He restores, confirms, strengthens,
and establishes me.

My God has spoken, this I know.
Therefore, I will not die but live,
for this storm shall pass.

Amen.

56

How often do I eagerly await the empty promises
of this life—
pursuing that which will surely fall,
those worthless treasures that disappear in an instant?
Yet, every one of those pursuits returns empty,
each one more disappointing than the last.

Until Jesus woke me up from my past,
He called me out of my grave.
In pain and suffering,
He gave me a pursuit everlasting—
one that does not return empty,
one that provides more with every attempt.
This is a pursuit worth chasing in this life,
the only one.

For all other pursuits return empty.

I was cast down;
all that I had was taken away from me.
I was struck down right where I stood;
I could not take another step.
Every moment became pain,
even my rest became a burden.
I was appalled at my reflection;
I kept my eyes fastened to that which was behind me.
I was overcome to the point of no emotion;

I had no tears to give.
Desperately, I reached out to this world,
and it left me to wither and rot.

But . . .
the God of Jacob took hold of me.
In chaos,
He saw my heart;
in despair,
He saw me through.
Although I continued to curse my Father,
He was a shield around me.
The waves of pain crashed against me,
yet my God never abandoned me.
All that I knew disappeared before me,
yet the Lord never let me go.

Why would I ever turn my back on this God?

Brothers and sisters,
why would we ever long for anything else?

Amen.

57

One cannot have faith without humility.
For without humility,
there is no need for faith,
no purpose for a Savior.

For this is why faith dies out
when life is easy—
why belief becomes dull
when days are filled with safety.

Humility admits that a gap exists
between who one is and what one deserves.
It causes the soul to confess
that this gap is impossibly distant.
Faith becomes the only option;
ultimately urgent.

Consider who you are today.
Consider your desires.
What exists in that place?

I am impossibly prideful,
my mind knows nothing of humility.
My deepest being desperately craves control,
I know little of what I deserve.

Amen.

58

Every piece of my body cries
    out for strength,
I can hardly hold myself up.
If my strength were my
    only hope,
it would not be long before I
    failed.

So in my emptiness,
let my wounds rejoice.
In my exhaustion,
let my spirit sing.
For I do not need to rely on
    myself for healing,
I am not on my own.
My God reigns in my
    weakness;
He is strong,
though I am not.
Therefore, let me be grateful
    in my wanting,
for in it,
I know my God must be.

A strength far greater exists,
a depth that does not succumb
    to circumstances.

In this place,
there is only room for God.
There is no space for pride,
no place for a self-
    righteous mind,
no room for personal desires.
Here, in this place,
there is but one strength,
the strength of the Lord.

Therefore, O Father,
remove me of myself.
Strip away my arrogance,
cast out my pride,
so there is only room for You.
Be my truth,
strengthen me according to
    Your mercy.
Do all that is necessary,
for You alone are my rock and
    my refuge.
It cannot be any other way.

I will put my trust in You,
or else my life should cease to
    go on.

Amen.

59

Woe is me,
I am overflowing with pride.
I cannot accept forgiveness,
for I am one who cannot extend forgiveness.
I cannot dwell in mercy and grace,
for I actively seek bitterness and resentment.

Therefore,
how can I receive that which I do not give?
How can I accept that which I do not pursue?

I cannot.

Father, I have a heart of stone.
All of my days are filled with indignation,
I obsess over the flaws that I seek.
I am consumed by my own self-sufficiency,
I am fooled by my pride.
For I am nothing but broken,
I am far from whole.
Yet You speak to me,
You seek me still.

Amen.

60

I am nothing if not weak,
I am empty on my own,
I cannot bear the weight of my suffering.
The evil of this world wears me down,
I have nothing to gain from it.
It has left me broken and destitute,
it smiles at the pain surrounding me.
Why, O soul, do you seek peace in this world?
Why, O spirit, do you seek truth in this place?
For all this world has,
all it can give,
is never enough.

Amen.

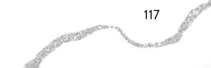

61

Who am I apart from my pain?
What can I do apart from my burden?
For I no longer see peace,
I forget the feeling of contentment.
What am I without my suffering?

My burden has become my comfort,
my pain is a close companion.
In my brokenness,
I have found escape;
I cannot see beyond this place.
I have turned my world upside down seeking to be made well,
yet my suffering persists.
I lament my place in this universe,
my days are full of wandering.

How sinister is the outward deception of strength
when sickness rages like a fire within me.
How cruel the ways of the evil one,
for he has made the eyes of others blind to my hurt.

Perhaps this is the greatest threat to my existence,
the fatigue of knowing
not a single soul understands.

I am certain that I no longer understand the simplest things in life,
basic is now complex.

O Lord, I have lost all sense,
I have questioned so much that I no longer live.
Rather, I sit and watch morning become evening,
days become weeks,
time is anything but linear.

Rid me of my doubt, O God,
root out the evil buried deep within me.
For generations,
You have delivered Your children;
will I be the first You will not?
Forgive me,
for the present overwhelms me.
It blinds me of the future,
it causes me to forget the past.

What all-knowing, perfect Creator
would waste such an unimaginable story?
For I have known more pain than joy,
more trauma than freedom,
more suffering than solidity.

That is why
I am ordained to change this world.

Amen.

62

I have fallen victim to
misunderstanding Your
magnitude, O Father.
Lulled to sleep by human
limitations,
You, O Lord, have become
small to me—
to my life
my need
my healing.
I fail to understand how much
You care for me.

Though I am small,
You give me Your undivided
attention.
Though I am sinful,
You hear my every word.
Though I am one of many,
I am once in an eternity to You.

How precious
is Your undivided attention.
How magnificent
is Your never-ending grace.
How bountiful
is Your earnestness to be
miraculous.

I considered myself
undeserving,
too focused on words,
distracted by voices,
ignoring Your touch.

Woe is me, Good Father,
yet I remain the apple of
Your eye.
I am not fit to live,
yet I am made in Your image.

Reignite a fire in me,
one that burns with belief.
Restore a confidence in me,
one that is fueled by faith.

You are not a bystander or
spectator,
You are the Lifeblood,
the very Source—
unmistakable, indescribable.
You will see to my victory.

Amen.

PART 7

FROM

RESILIENCE

TO

STRENGTH

We . . .
decide to carry on
put one foot in front of the other
refuse to give in
which leads to . . .
resilience.

It is God who arms me with strength and
keeps my way secure. . . . He trains my hands
for battle; my arms can bend a bow of bronze.
(2 Samuel 22:33, 35)

He . . .
who delights in blessing His children
who sees the conviction in our hearts
who uplifts the humble
calls us into . . .
the strength of His Spirit.

63

I have been blind.
My ears listened,
but they did not hear.
My mouth spoke,
but my words withered with the wind.

But . . .
now my eyes see,
and my ears hear.
Let my lips proclaim wisdom that takes hold in the soil,
its roots deeply woven into the earth.

Make my fear my greatest understanding,
for fear of You brings knowledge and righteousness.
It brings me low,
makes my knees give way
to the splendor,
the power,
the majesty,
of the Lord God in Heaven.

Forgive me, O Father,
in Your grace,
comfort me.
Make me strong again in your presence,
for from this truth I will never depart.

Amen.

64

Father,
You will not let me bear alone a weight I
    cannot handle.
You will not allow death to be my end today.

You have set apart a path for me here,
of which I do not know,
for I cannot see.
But when that day comes,
my joy will be a melody in Your courts.
My spirit will overflow with gratitude,
and I will not turn back.

For in the evening,
You lay my head down,
and in the morning,
Your grace sustains me when I rise.
On that day,
You will declare healing,
comfort will descend on high like rain.
You will deliver me from the clutches of death,
and I will see Your face like the sun that shines.

Do not hide Your face,
do not lower Your voice;
be near.
Be my I Am,
be my King.
Be my ever-present,
be my breath.
Be my morning and my evening,
be my joy and my truth.

Fill my cup,
strengthen my feet beneath me.
Look on me with grace,
forgive me with Your kindness.
Know in me what the eye cannot see,
and the ear cannot hear.

For I am nothing—
not a human,
not a body, mind, or soul—
I am nothing,
if I am not Yours.

Amen.

65

The mind of humanity is weak;
I am a human.

I seek contentment,
I pursue peace,
yet I do not fear the Lord;
I fear the world.
I will never be content,
peace will never be my
    companion,
unless I fear the Lord,
not the world.

The one who seeks fulfillment
    in this life
has not known suffering.
Those who fill their days
    chasing success
do not know truth.
Those who pursue fame and
    fortune
do not know peace.

My Father in Heaven,
may Your praise be on my lips.
My King and my Comfort,
may Your name alone be
    hallowed.
Remove my selfish will from
    before me,
in its place bring Your Spirit of
    truth.

Instill Your righteousness
    in me,
be the overflow of my cup.
If on this day
I lose more of myself and gain
    more of You,
my soul will rejoice.

Let it be so.

Amen.

66

Will I ever rise again?
Will peace be my companion once more?

O God, my God,
see this torment that surrounds me.
Look on me with forgiveness,
rescue me with your salvation.
No longer do I pray for healing,
but for a miracle.

For I know nothing apart from You,
and in this,
my life was made complete.
I will not waste away,
I will be victorious in Your grace,
conqueror in Your mercy.
You will establish me for Your kingdom,
I will run and not grow weary.

Make my joy complete,
because only in You will I have complete joy.
Then, I will sing Your praise,
I will walk the path You established before me.

Praise be to God Almighty;
He has done a miracle in me today.

Amen.

67

My spirit and my body are strangers,
they are foreigners to each other.
My spirit says *Go,*
but my body cannot move.
My spirit says *Peace alone,*
but my body trembles with fear.
My spirit says *This pain is ending,*
but my body is paralyzed by suffering.
Peace is a distant memory,
I have no rest.

My body despises me,
it sees me as its enemy,
it does not hold back.

Conquer my body,
just as You conquered my spirit.
Deliver me from this constant pain,
just as You delivered me from my sin.
Restore my body to wholeness,
just as You restored my soul to eternity.
Establish the work of my hands,
just as You established Your will in my heart.

Amen.

68

Father, You wove me together
until I was pleasing in your sight.

Then I ran from You.

My life was my own,
I took it for myself and abandoned Your truth.
I hid in every corner,
every dark place was my home.
I could not stand before You,
Your Word was foreign to me.

In my moment of despair,
my time of complete suffering and destruction,
You found me.
You forced me to look upon Your face;
I lay before You with fear and trembling.

Now I see my life was never my own.
Every corner, every dark place,
You were there.
Your hand was over me,
Your angels surrounded me.
For You have plans for me.

In Your goodness, You kept me.

Amen.

69

It is by the grace of God
that I am standing.
It is by His redemption alone
that I have breath.

For I have seen the face of death,
I have looked into the eyes of evil.
The enemy has been near in every affliction,
his blade has covered my body in scars.
Yet here I stand,
for this there is but one reason:
my heavenly Father demands to have me.

Therefore, no longer will I hide my scars in shame,
no longer will fear grip my spirit.
I will trust in the name of the Lord,
for it is the only Name that gives life.
Be my portion, Jesus;
uphold me, loving Father.
The time has come
for Your name to be established on my lips,
Your power to be made known through my hands.

Lift me up from the pit,
rescue me from the jaws of death.
Break the chains that hold me,
set me free from the chaos surrounding me.
You alone, Father, can restore me,
in Your strength alone,
I will be well.
Overcome the death that circles,
pull me out of the suffering that grips me.

Declare victory over Your child;
drive out evil from this place,
for it has been welcome far too long.
I will find no rest until I am established in You,
this I know.

Deliver me, my God and Conqueror;
I will praise Your name forever.
Establish goodness in this home;
let all generations praise the Lord,
now and forever,
for the mercy of the Lord endures forever.

Amen.

70

Steady the ship of my anxiety,
  O Lord,
calm the storm that rages
  against me.
In the morning,
I look to You,
For I know that You are
  setting my feet on solid
  ground;
You are renewing my soul.

Therefore, let me walk with
  power,
turn my eyes to look upon
  Your face.
Pick me up,
lead me in the ways of the
  upright,
set my feet on the path of life.
For Your burden is easy,
and Your yoke is light.

You have determined my steps
  before me,
in grace
You have commanded my spirit.
What, then, can stand
  against me?

For I have seen the darkness of
  doubt,
the frozen embrace of pain has
  suffocated me.
Yet in my darkest moment,
Your light broke through.
It overwhelmed my spirit,
it brought warmth to my soul.

Praise be to the God of
  providence.

For not a tree falls in the forest
without Your command.
Not a breath is taken
without Your permission.
The wind does now blow,
the sun does not shine,
without Your voice.

Amen.

71

My God overcomes,
my God is bigger,
my God is stronger.
Therefore, I will put my trust in Him,
for trust in myself will surely fail.

I have lived unto myself,
and I have suffered for it.
I know pain,
I dwell with suffering.
Trauma awaits me at every turn,
abuse has demanded to have my soul.
Yet, by the grace of God,
I am on my knees today.
Because of the mercy of Him who knows
    nothing else,
there is breath in my lungs.
The moment my faith leaves me behind
is the moment I will no longer live.
Father, I cannot see the light,
the darkness is insurmountable.
Long has the enemy dwelled in my presence,
his eyes desire to see me fall.
He has blinded me to the power of my God,
he longs to fill my mind with lies.

Overcome this fear,
root out my anxiety.
Look on me with power,
call me into Your presence.
Lift me out of my misery,
restore my trembling soul.
Draw me out of darkness,
set me into Your light.

Do not delay any longer,
look upon me here and now.
Have mercy on my empty spirit,
deliver me from this desolate wasteland.
Cast me into the land of promises,
set my feet on the shores of freedom.
I will not know life of my own,
Your will alone is my portion forever.

You, my God, can overcome;
You, O Father, can do all things.
Cause my weary heart to believe, merciful Lord,
deliver me into Your promises.
I will go.

Amen.

72

Speak, O Lord,
do not withhold a word
   from me.

I Am who I Am.
I am He who created the
   heavens and the earth,
He who rose up all that is
   within it.
I am He who created man and
   woman,
He who formed you with
   intimate detail.
Look and see,
I am He who created the stars in
   the sky,
the universe in its majesty.
I am God,
He who was before there was
   nothing,
He who will stand for eternity.
I am Creator, boundless
   Creator,
My might has no limit,
it will not end.

I am the Lord your God.
You cannot fathom what you
   cannot see,
you cannot know what is foreign
   to you.
Look and see,
your Creator commands you to
   look and see.
My creation is intricate,
each piece has been wonderfully
   spoken.
Although the shadows of sin grow,
My beauty persists in every shade.

O child, creation of mine,
you are the most personal of
   them all.
Look and see,
every creature,
every plant,
every place,
it all belongs to Me.
Among everything,
there is no creation like you, O
   child.
Among the stars in the sky,
within the galaxies and the
   universe,
there is none like you.

Where can you go
that I am not there already?
What darkness exists
that I have not faced and
  overcome?
O you of little faith,
do you hear Me?
Can you fathom the power of
  My right hand,
or the splendor of My voice?
Do you see outside of time,
can you hold the planets in your
  palm?

Look around and see, O child,
look at me.
I am who I am,
and you are My beloved.
Go forward with faith,
do not look back again.
Be healed by trusting your
  Father.
Do not be afraid,
do not withhold;
I am He who created you,
He who walks beside you.

Your breath gives me life,
  O God,
Your Word sets me free.

Amen.

73

Father, God,
cause me to submit all of my ways to You.
Time and time again,
I stumble and fall.
Yet I know with all my heart,
I cannot be apart from You.
Surely, I know
I cannot stand on my own,
I cannot walk without Your guidance.
So here I am,
on my knees before Your throne.
And I ask of You, O God,
to equip me for Your purposes.
I pray that You send me forth
to do Your will.

O mind, why do you fear?
O soul, why do you hold back?

God, my Creator,
wash me clean as I am reborn.
Empty me of the evil in my bones,
that I might be laid out before You.
No longer can I be without You,
I condemn my body of flesh and brittle waste.
Give me a new body, O God,
instill Your Spirit within a new temple!

Out with the old, in with the new,
I do not wish to keep an ounce of myself.
Rid me of the toxic sinfulness that rips into my flesh,
condemn the evil that gnaws at my bones.

Least qualified,
most broken and flawed,
here I stand.
Least worthy,
most weary and undeserving,
here I stand.
Give me life everlasting,
send me where I am needed for Your kingdom.
Give me faith unshakeable,
beckon me into healing and life eternal.

Dissolve my fears,
extinguish my selfish desires,
lead me to freedom's gate.

I am no longer dead,
for my cup runs over.
I am no longer sick,
for the Lord reigns within me.

I will go forth with faith, and not turn back.

Amen.

74

The sun is up,
the darkness has given into the morning light;
Your mercy is upon me.
Awaken my heart to Your truth,
open my eyes to Your Word;
I will gaze upon You.

Long have I wandered,
many days have passed,
but I will seek Your glory.

O Father, move in this place.
Make me aware of Your providence,
let me give in to Your ways.
Cause me to pursue Your will,
with every ounce of intention.
Give me Your wisdom
as I seek a life of servanthood.

I cannot be still.

I am a wild animal
locked in a cage;
set me free.
But, my God,
only to do Your will.
I refuse to seek myself.

Strike me down,
destroy my life,
if I desire to keep it.

Mighty and wonderful Creator,
You have plans to prosper me.
Good and faithful God,
You will establish the work of my hands.
Loving Father,
You will not let Your child stray.

Therefore,
break the chains that hold me.
Fear,
worry,
pride—
let them fall away.

Set me free with power,
with power and joy,
that I may dwell in Your presence,
that I may further Your kingdom.

Let it be.

Amen.

75

I need healing, O God,
You are my healer.

I need forgiveness, O God,
forgive my sins.

I need hope, O God,
give me hope.

I need peace, O God,
be my peace.

I need faith, O God,
heal me with faith.

I need love, O God,
please give me love.

Do not let evil prevail, O Lord,
You will conquer.

Do not let anger control me, O Lord,
You will overcome.

Do not let fear destroy me, O Lord,
You will not lose.

Do not let me wither, O Lord,
You will love.

I am Your beloved, O Father,
I will prevail.

I am Your warrior, O Father,
I have victory.

I am Your servant, O Father,
I have purpose.

I am a sinner, O Father,
set me free.

I am so broken, O Father,
please heal me.

I am Your creation, O Father,
I am Your child.

In this world I am nothing,
in this world I have nothing,
but, at Your feet, O God,
I have all things.

Amen.

PART 8

FROM

REDEMPTION

TO

DELIVERANCE

We . . .
find gratitude in our hardship
find hope in our suffering
find freedom in our afflictions
which leads to . . .
redemption.

I pursued my enemies and crushed them; I
did not turn back till they were destroyed. . . .
You armed me with strength for battle; You
humbled my adversaries before me.
(2 Samuel 22:38, 40)

He . . .
who desires to be the joy of our hearts
who longs to be our foundation
who rejoices in our thanksgiving
calls us into . . .
deliverance from darkness.

76

My King.
My steps had grown unsteady,
my feet began to slip.
For I was intent on the potential of the future,
infatuated with the freedom of the past.
Yet, all the while,
my eyes did not consider the present.

Replace the sand with rock,
bring praising hands instead of shackled wrists.
Hold me close to You,
so that all I see is Your tender love and mercy,
Your awesome power and might.
Let every breath be praise to You,
fill my cup with joy and gratitude.

Amen.

77

Under rocks and within every nook,
I have searched for identity.
Places high and low,
I have gone to feel something.
What was I after?
What did my soul long to see?
For what I found was emptiness,
loss,
darkness.

Yet,
You pursued me.

Under rocks and within every nook,
You pursued me until my identity was
    rooted in You.
Places high and low,
You were there to give me peace.
Why did You wait?
Why did You long to have my soul?

Why did You seek me when I ran?
For You care for Your flock, O Shepherd,
every one.

And,
You found me.

In my deepest loss, my truest pain,
You reached out to me.
In my darkest place,
there You came to find me.

My soul longs to be with You,
my body bears the scars from when I ran from You.
Your power is my breath,
Your grace is my well-being.
Surely Your mercy and goodness will follow me
all the days of my life.

Amen.

78

I cannot stand righteous in the courts of heaven.
I cannot present a single defense
that could be upheld by the God of the universe.
If I pursued a case for myself,
it would quickly be thrown out.
I have no ability to stand on my own two feet,
nothing in me is untouched by sin.
These things I know for certain.

If my only hope was to have more good than bad,
more purity than evil,
I would surely spend eternity in the pit.
This I know to be true:
that a perfect God could not justify my soul by
    works alone.
A holy, blameless Creator would not take me in,
for my ways are far from perfect.

How, then, can I enter the Kingdom of Forever?
How can I be justified, redeemed, forgiven?
How can the case against me be dropped?
There is but one option.

A gift from the Judge on high,
a perfect trade-off—
one who lived and breathed
exactly the opposite of me.

One without a sinful bone in His body;
One without a single charge against Him;
One with complete and total purity of mind,
    spirit, and body.
This gift of a sacrifice,
one of a perfect life,
a perfect death,
a perfect resurrection.
The only One who deserved eternal life,
yet was unjustly sentenced to death.

Why this?
Why is this the only way?
Because I can be justified by faith, not by works.
Because I can now plead guilty,
yet the charges are dropped against me.

For the Creator always desired
to be perfectly connected to the creation,
but sin stood in the way.
Yet when the perfect sacrifice is received,
this impurity is washed away with salvation.

Creator can once again dwell with creation.

Amen.

79

We are foolish,
we are broken.
We are ignorant,
we are ill-spoken.

We are prideful,
we are hopeless.
We are corrupt,
but we are still *chosen*.

God is wise,
God is whole.
God is righteous,
God is full.

God is humble,
God is hope.
God is perfect,
God is on the throne.

Let us return to dust and ashes
if we forget.

Amen.

80

Father, forgive me.

For I envy those who have more than I do.
I am filled with bitterness toward You.
I do not trust You with all of my heart,
    mind, soul, and strength.
I do not cast my anxieties on You.
Forgive me for being deceived by the enemy,
for filling my own mind with lies.
For failing to prepare for battle,
for avoiding my sin.
For being quick to anger,
for failing to allow others into my suffering.
For being timid, afraid, and weak-minded,
for loving sin and complacency.

I am a sinner.

I will praise my God,
for He has forgiven me.

Amen.

81

I will trust in the Lord.
I will drive out evil,
I will command healing by His Spirit,
and in His name.
He is my Daily Bread,
my portion and my cup forever.
I will be made well in the name of the Almighty,
through the Lamb of God seated at His right hand.

Holy Spirit, drive out this evil from me.
Come, take its place within me.
For the Lord is my Healer;
He restores my soul.

No longer will I be under the command of evil,
no longer am I chained by suffering.
For my God is greater than these.

God, let Your light drive out this darkness,
let Your presence make evil scatter.
For it cannot be where You are.

Declare it in this moment of attack;
crush my enemy with Your hand,
that Your powerful name would be known.

Amen.

82

The only freedom I knew
was freedom in the world.
So, freedom is something I never knew.

The only life I knew
was life in the world.
So, life is something I never knew.

The only joy I knew
was joy in the world.
So, joy is something I never knew.

And then,
the world cast me down.
It abused me and destroyed my body.
It poisoned my mind,
left me for dead.

But,
my God demanded to have me.
In complete darkness,
I was given the light of truth.
In utter despair,
I was given salvation.

Now I know,
my only freedom is in God's forgiveness,
my only life is in the death of myself,
my only joy is in the eternity of salvation.

Although I am still weak,
as my body fights against me,
and my mind loses its identity,
I have life forevermore.

For if this pain has given me eternity with
the Creator,
I will choose it from this day until my last.

Amen.

83

I have sought a life of comfort and ease.
One that is filled with expectation,
a picture of normality and stability.
However, I see the foolishness of this desire,
the deception of its lies and distractions.
For this life is no life at all.

Rather, it is a slow death,
a flame that gradually fades,
until its memory is empty and no more—
fool's gold.

Why, brothers and sisters,
do we seek a life that slowly fades into
    nothingness?
Why, brothers and sisters,
do we desire a life of fleeting purpose and
    emptiness?

Do we not know that in a moment,
we could breathe our last breath?
That wind and rain could sweep away all
    that we have?

We know nothing of truth,
we are consumed by deception and
   distraction.
False security is our deepest desire,
pride is our truest companion.

Our pursuit in this life
is in that which will be forgotten the
   moment we are no more.
How trivial is our coming and going,
how shallow is our understanding.

From the moment we take our first breath,
our motive is to accumulate everything
   that will disappear.
Let us turn from our foolishness,
let us pursue that which will never perish.

Amen.

8 4

What does the Lord ask of me?
What does He want from me?

Far too long I have imposed my will on
    the Lord,
for I desire the things of this world.
Yet, all can be taken from me,
except my God.
In a moment,
the things of this life can disappear,
except my God.
Though still I seek what the world can
    give me,
empty-handed it leaves me.

Father, empower me to abandon this
    foolish hope,
and give me more of You.
Replace my desires of this world,
with an ever-growing obsession for You.
Overwhelm my spirit,
overcome my desperate need to be someone.
Instead,
let me cling to being Your child.
Cause Your Holy Spirit to descend upon
    every part of me,
do not leave any stone unturned.

O dear brothers and sisters,
return to He who knows you best.
The more you seek in this world,
the darker it becomes.
The more you desire to satisfy yourself,
the emptier you will be.
You have a Father,
a perfect and holy King.
He desires to be with you,
He longs to see you return home.

I will abandon my pursuits in this world, O Lord;
I refuse to take another step
if I am not first obsessed with Jesus.
Cause my heart to stop beating,
keep air from my lungs,
if I am not first a beloved child of God.

Let my every breath be praise,
let every moment be worship.
If I am nothing else,
let me rejoice that I am Yours.

Amen.

85

I do not know the ways of
the Lord,
I do not see the plans of the
Father.
I cannot fathom the mercy of
the King,
nor understand the
boundlessness of His love.

The ways of the Lord are
faultless;
He is mighty in wonder,
great in His ways.

The Lord gives,
and the Lord takes.
The Almighty God raises,
and He puts to rest.
Nothing is apart from His
sight.
Therefore, I will rejoice in His
mercy.

In the oceans of His grace,
I am free.
I will not be bound by this
world—
sickness
loss
pain
suffering
even death—
but in everything,
I have been set free.

For His ways are good,
His justice commands
my soul.
This place is not my home,
it will forever let me down.
Broken
corrupt
evil—
I long for heaven.

O Father,
how weak is my mind!
Capture my gaze,
fix my eyes on You;
You will not let me down.
Take away all that I have,
remove my life from in front
    of me
if it makes me Your child.
Cause my body to wither,
to shrivel and shake,
if I seek to keep my life in this
    world.
Separate me from any
    distraction,
abolish any semblance of
    entitlement,
so that I can be Yours.

Why, O my soul, have you
    held onto this life?
I will cast myself into the dirt
to be reborn in Christ.
Put this body of sin to death,
nail it to the cross of separation,
so that I can be known by You.

O, how worth it will it be,
a fullness everlasting,
when not a single piece of me
    remains,
and the Spirit of God lives
    in me.

Amen.

86

You are a jealous God.

Creator of all things,
mighty and intricate,
You are a magnificent God.

Provider of all things,
big and small,
You are a sovereign God.

Ruler of all things,
yesterday, today, and tomorrow,
You are an infinite God.

Filled with many worries,
complex and simple,
I am a weak child.

Foolishly seeking control,
every little detail,
I am a hopeless child.

Blown by the wind,
strong and gentle,
I am a distracted child.

You are a jealous God,
I am a sinful child.

Intimately, uniquely, wonderfully,
You made me.
Yet, in an instant,
I turn my back on You.

Bountifully, graciously, patiently,
You give me all things.
Yet, in a moment,
I give in to endless sin.

You are jealous,
because I am a fool.

Do not give up on me, O Father,
You never will.

Forgive me of my sin, O God,
You always will.

I will seek to bring You joy,
in Your presence I will dwell.
I will be more like You.

Amen.

87

I am blind to Your truth,
ignorant to Your teaching,
empty of Your commands.

I run from Your direction,
then curse Your name violently.
I condemn Your sovereignty,
believing that I know better.

In my immeasurable pride,
You humbled me.

You inherited my pain,
You brought me low;
now I see Your face.
You are a God of patience,
delivering me out of self-reliance.
Make me aware of my sin,
and I will spend my days fighting temptation.

God of all creation,
make me sober-minded and watchful.
Deliver me from self-righteousness,
make me more like Your Son.

For I may be a sinner,
broken and foolish,
but I am still loved unconditionally.

There is no freedom such as this,
no joy that compares,
to the embrace of my heavenly Father.

In Him,
there is truth.
With Him,
there is no fear.
At His feet,
I am set free.

Nothing can compare.

You are my peace.
You are my identity.
You are my forgiveness.
You are my hope.

I am nothing apart from You—
how wonderful.

Amen.

8 8

How can we stand in Your presence, O God?
Constantly,
we depart from You.
Without thought,
we turn from You.
Disobedience is our most consistent quality.

Inclined to sin,
we ignore our greatest treasure.
Cause us, O God,
to know better.
To treasure You and Your Word,
obeying Your commands,
for freedom is at Your feet.

Patiently,
You wait.
As a stern yet tender Father,
You wait.

Let us turn from our ways, brothers and sisters,
turn!
Though our God is full of forgiveness,
He cannot be mocked.
Let us return to Him,
abandon our pride and return.

There is no other love like this,
the love of our Maker.
There is no other redemption like this,
the redemption of our Father.

Let us consider our sin,
remember our brokenness,
call to mind every burden.
Cast it all on the Lord,
lay it down at His feet.
He is able,
willing,
waiting
to pour out His love.

Why would we stand in the presence
of any other?
There is no one like You.

Amen.

PART 9

FROM
PRAISE TO
ADOPTION

We ...
are renewed by faith
are redeemed by God's love
are given an ultimate identity
which leads to ...
a life of praise.

Therefore I will praise you, LORD, among the
nations; I will sing the praises of your name.
(2 Samuel 22:50)

He ...
who treasures His sons and daughters
who is glorified in our faith
who is worthy of all things
calls us into ...
an eternal adoption.

89

O Lord,
I will praise Your name.
Praise Your name here on earth,
as it is in heaven.
May Your name be known throughout
the earth,
bless us so that it may be so.
Bless us as children who fear You alone,
for it is Your name that is above all others.

Equip these hands,
move this body,
fix these eyes
on You and Your truth alone.

Let Your name be on my lips,
and Your truth be written in my heart.
For You, O God, are power;
You, O God, are righteousness;
You, O God, are everlasting;
You, O God, are alone on the throne.

I call to You, O Father,
save me.

Bring healing upon this weary soul,
that I might praise Your grace.

Cast this evil from my presence, Father,
claim victory and power over it.
Disperse its hold on my body,
and free me from its grasp.

Let Your power be proclaimed
here and now,
and Your praise I will sing until I am
no more.

Amen.

90

The sun and stars are Your workmanship, O Lord,
the skies above are a canvas of Your magnitude.

With a word,
the heavens pour out rain,
giving life to all.
In a moment the rain stops,
and the sun shines again.

The land trembles at the thunder,
which roars down on the earth.
The lightning illuminates all that we see,
and in a moment it disappears at Your command.

You are God of the universe.
The galaxies and planets within,
they reveal an endless glimpse into Your handiwork.
You are God of all.

Praise His name, O earth,
shout at His magnificent wonder.
Fear the Lord our God,
tremble at His mighty power.
For in the same moment that He wipes away,
He restores again those who are righteous.

I lift up my voice,
I have nothing else to give
but a humble heart and a broken spirit.

Restore my soul, O God,
look on me with kindness.

Give me victory,
rescue me from death.

I will praise Your name forever.

Amen.

91

Though my body withers away,
my Redeemer lives,
and I will see His face.
I will look upon my Savior and rejoice,
my soul will shout for victory.

He has set my feet on solid ground,
He has shown His goodness to me.
He has fought for the life of His beloved,
He has saved me from death.

Confirm Your will for me, O God,
restore salvation in my body once again.
Strengthen the armor of the Almighty around me,
the heavenly host over me,
establish my hands as a servant for Your kingdom.

For my life is Yours alone;
I would have no will if it were not.
Therefore, I will boast that You conquered my life,
that You are victorious within me.
I will cry tears of joy that my sin is forgiven,
I will shout Your name until my voice is gone.

For You have done the impossible,
You have overcome what was insurmountable.
You redeemed the heart of a wretch,
You washed clean the spirit of a born sinner.

How could I ever claim a life of my own?

When in Your presence alone,
I am alive.
When subject to Your perfect ways,
I am free.
When at Your right hand,
I have pleasures forevermore.

You have done the unimaginable:
made perfect that which is wholly imperfect.

Shout for joy to the Lord our God!

Amen.

92

Let my prayer come before the Lord of glory.
May my words fill Your presence with a pleasing aroma.

O my lips, speak humbly to the King of kings;
may my tongue bring truth to the Father.
For You have beckoned my soul to You,
so my soul sings praise,
because the God of the universe knows me.

I have listened to your prayers, O child,
I have known your suffering and heard your cry.
You have pursued that which is not for you,
that which belongs to Me.
You have run from Me,
but I never lost sight of you for a moment.
Many sought to steal your joy,
but My mercy was ever upon you.

I will praise the Lord,
for He delivered me from death.

Amen.

93

Tender and powerful,
kind and mighty,
humble and divine,
You are the only God.

A wholly perfect juxtaposition,
perfect God and perfect man,
this is the only God.

Rightful Judge,
yet full of mercy,
intimate Creator,
yet expansive in knowledge,
this is the only God.

For I am just a human:
desperate and lowly,
coldhearted and weak,
selfish and unable,
prideful and broken,
my only choice is this God.

A wholly imperfect body
    and soul,
imperfect flesh and imperfect
    desires,
my only choice is this God.

Destined for death,
yet full of expectation,
constantly hiding,
yet obsessed with myself,
my only option is this God.

Therefore,
I cannot stand,
so I will kneel.
I cannot hold my head high,
so I will bow.
I cannot control a thing,
so I will submit.
I cannot satisfy myself,
so I will follow You.
I cannot live forever,
so I will put my faith in You.

This God,
my God.
The only God.

Amen.

94

Today is brand-new.
The clouds have passed,
the sun rises and shines bright.
The gentle strength of grace has set me free.
If forgiveness reigns,
my chains no longer exist.
The miracle of love washes over me,
nothing can be hidden from the God of providence.

Therefore, I fall down in worship;
tears of loss are replaced with tears of victory.
What was meant for harm,
God is making for good.
For the enemy made me a victim,
but the Lord makes me a survivor.
No longer will I take shelter in my suffering;
I will not be a prisoner to my pain.
Rather, by the ultimate sacrifice of love,
I will be victorious.

I do not wish to live without my God,
surely my life would be chaos and destruction.
For I have wandered meaninglessly,
I have been taken by the current of complacency,
and my life was certain to be death.
I struck out on my own;
I pursued a life for my sake,
and I found no purpose to carry on.

Therefore, I will choose to be a survivor,
because my God died on the cross for me.
I will choose the way of life,
because my Father gives me breath.
I will have my victory,
because the Spirit of the Lord does not lose.

I have returned to You, O God;
receive me in my brokenness.
Show me the way to victory;
lead me down the path to eternity.
Make me Yours,
or do not give me another breath.

Amen.

95

Praise!
Praise be unto Him,
in the midst of suffering.
Praise His holy name,
because of the pain.

Because of my afflictions,
I will praise You relentlessly.
Because of this hurt,
I will depend on You unceasingly.
Because nothing else will satisfy my longing,
I will worship you fiercely.

I will shout for joy,
for trials bring me closer to Jesus.

Amen.

O mighty God,
You cannot be stopped.
You are a tidal wave of majesty,
a tornado of power;
there is none like You.

In a moment,
I am both overwhelmed at Your magnitude,
and underwhelmed by my response.
For I lack proper understanding,
I fail to see Your glory.

O intimate Creator,
Your love is astounding.
You are an ocean of grace,
a storm of mercy;
there is nothing like You.

In the midst of persecution,
I see the beauty of Your providence,
and the wonders of Your movement.
For often I seek my own way,
but Your plans cannot be thwarted.

Amen.

97

Praise the Father,
for He created you and me.
Praise the Son,
for He died our death.
Withstanding the wrath of God,
in a moment of separation,
Jesus died for you and me.
Praise the Spirit,
for He is alive in us today.

O you people, wake up!
See what the Lord has done for you,
be changed and take heart.
Do not be fools,
do not be indifferent,
nothing else matters but this.

Read His Word,
it is written for you.
Obey His commands,
they are freedom for you.
Love His people,
this is joy for you.
Serve His kingdom,
inherit eternal life,
this is everything for you.

Amen.

98

Father,
guide my tongue.
Bring peace to my mind.
Give strength to my body.
Convict my heart.

I will obey Your commands.
I will fear You.
I will serve You.
I will walk in obedience,
loving You above all else.

Forgive me of my sin,
make me well.

Amen.

99

O, that I might live a life
worthy of the Messiah—
to walk like Him,
to talk like Him,
to be His image bearer.

Although impossible,
this is my life's pursuit,
a goal I will never achieve,
yet a cause worth living for,
worth dying for—
knowing I will never be free in this life,
and finding freedom in that truth.

What more could I want?
What else can I seek,
but the grace and the truth,
the light of life,
He who conquered death?

Forgiveness is in the scars on Your hands,
hope is found at the empty tomb.
I have peace,
knowing I am saved by Your death,
though I do not deserve it.
I have conviction,
knowing I am called by You.

No one compares to You,
almighty Savior.
Yet,
You cry with me,
You hurt by my side,
You love my joy.

Because of this,
I will praise You.
I will worship You
in action and in thought;
I will glorify Your name.

Son of God,
Son of Man,
there is no one like You.

Praise His name.

Amen.

100

O Father,
There are few things I know for certain:
You are almighty and all-powerful;
You are all-loving and forgiving;
You care about me to an extent
I cannot fathom,
and I am completely helpless,
and undeserving by my own accord.

Search my heart,
and know that I desire You.
Teach me to understand Your truth,
to seek righteousness,
and to gain wisdom.
Forgive my constant sinful nature,
and restore me until my last breath,
for Your Names' sake.

Amen.

In Closing

In crisis,
the Lord is my safety.
His Word is my light,
His presence is my comfort.

I call out to the Lord in trouble,
knowing He will answer me.
He listens,
earnestly waiting to respond to His children.

With power and mercy,
the Lord speaks to His beloved.
With grace and forgiveness,
He shows us truth.
Suffering brings me to my knees,
as grief swallows me whole.
But God is my rescue,
He will not let me go.

Destruction clouds my mind,
it makes me wander without hope.
Yet the Lord calls me to obedience,
His Word makes my path straight.

When pain threatens my inmost being,
bringing me to the depths of despair,
the blood of the Lamb gives me resilience.

Resilience gives way to life,
I will trust in the Lord for strength;
the Spirit of God is my endurance.

Perseverance becomes my identity,
the Father gives me purpose in my perspective.
Though the enemy seeks me still,
my foundation will never be broken.

I am redeemed in affliction,
for suffering brings me closer to Jesus.
I will praise His name in darkness,
I will never relent.

Amen.

A Final Charge

Hello, Friend.

Though I may not know your name, I am praying for you and thanking God for your life.

As you may have discovered through reading this book, I am not shy about the intense experiences of darkness we face in this life. We are bound together—painfully and wonderfully bound—by this experience of suffering. I have learned to honor this, rather than hide or suppress it, because I believe suffering is deserving of our honest, vulnerable, and biblically sound honor. After all, the Savior we worship was put on this earth to experience the ultimate suffering that, now, we never need to.

However, I must wholeheartedly inform you that our story does not end here. Our suffering does not end in suffering; our darkness does not end in darkness. You and I are being redeemed and restored with each passing moment until, one day soon, our ultimate victory will arrive. After all, our Savior did not remain in His tomb but for a brief moment, until He walked out and returned to His heavenly place at the right hand of the Father.

So, too, it will be for us.

In the end, every ounce of hurt will be eternally restored by our perfect Creator. Our day is coming. He is coming.

So, I want to offer you a final word of encouragement, an

all-encompassing summary of my desire to write this book and share it with you: suffer earnestly and hope earnestly. Press on in your afflictions—your grief, your pain, your loss, your darkness—and press on in faithful hope, in steadfast faith. In that spirit, I want to share together in one final prayer:

There is a day soon coming,
that every single one of my sorrows
will be redeemed,
and I will be restored.

Though it may never come
in this life,
it will undoubtedly come,
and joy will be mine.

If Your promises are true, O Lord,
I am content to live the rest of
   my days
in suffering;
for I know the prize that awaits me
in perseverance.

In every one of my afflictions,
draw near to me, Lord.
Strengthen my faith—
make me resilient
in my suffering,
not after it is through.

Fill my cup with the joy
of everlasting hope in You,
   O mighty God,
that I may persist in the battle,
and have the victory.

The day is fast approaching,
where light will swallow
   darkness whole,
and I will sit in my heavenly
   place.

Therefore,
with every passing moment,
I will fight—
standing firm in my faith,
steadfast in my obedience,
preparing to receive my
   eternal crown.

Amen.

Acknowledgments

It is impossible to properly thank and capture all the wonderful people and resources that made this book possible, but I will give it my best shot in the only way I know how:

To my beautiful bride, who saw me at my lowest and chose me still, thank you for setting yourself aside and remaining next to me even when I was giving you so little.

To my wonderful mom and dad, who wanted to take my pain and were instead forced to watch their son suffer, thank you for fighting so many battles on my behalf.

To my brother and sister (my best friends), who shared in every tear, hopeless moment, and wild inconvenience, thank you for giving me life-saving moments of laughter, joy, and hope.

To my extended family and friends, who opened their homes and hands to me, thank you for every seen and unseen support you provided for me.

To my newfound friends and family at HarperCollins, who supported this project from the very first moment, thank you for taking such a risk on an unproven outsider with a notebook.

To my dedicated agent Kathleen, who stepped in and saved me at the eleventh hour, thank you for believing in me and encouraging me to be an author.

To the saints David and Job, who I have not met but soon will, thank you for showing me how to suffer well and with the Lord.

To everyone else that played a uniquely vital role in my hardships and the production of this book: Laura, MacKenzie, Bonnie, Sabryna, Emily, Gunk Gunk, Chris and Lacey, Carissa, Brett and Hannah, Charlie, Malik, Daniel, Beth, Danielle, Brendan, Brent, and the wonderful community at Nashville Life Church, thank you.

Most importantly, to my Redeemer and Rescue, whose feet I am not worthy to clean, whose glory could not be captured even if I spent the rest of my life writing about it, thank You for saving my life.

About the Author

BEN LOCKE is a former collegiate soccer player, MBA graduate, and small business owner. Although he doesn't quite understand how and when it happened, Ben is also a writer and poet.

After chronic illness forced him to abandon his hopes of playing professional soccer, Ben dove headfirst into writing as a means of escape, expression, and faith. Without any agenda, he began journaling his exchanges and interactions with the Lord, often hunched over the side of his bed due to his illness. Now, Ben is inspiring the often-silenced voices of the sick, lost, lonely, and hopeless.

This honest pursuit, along with the unwavering support of his family, also led him to come forward about the sexual abuse he endured as a student-athlete. His unexpected discovery of the profound grace of God, combined with his intense experiences of pain and suffering, motivate him to speak with directness, write with vulnerability, and tell the story of the broken.

He recently launched an online journal called *Evensong*, which is a weekly writing shared with readers interested in communal prayer.